# Palliative Care in Nursing & Healthcare

# Palliative Care in Nursing & Healthcare

Michelle Brown

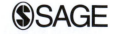

Los Angeles | London | New Delhi
Singapore | Washington DC

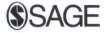

Los Angeles | London | New Delhi
Singapore | Washington DC

SAGE Publications Ltd
1 Oliver's Yard
55 City Road
London EC1Y 1SP

SAGE Publications Inc.
2455 Teller Road
Thousand Oaks, California 91320

SAGE Publications India Pvt Ltd
B 1/I 1 Mohan Cooperative Industrial Area
Mathura Road
New Delhi 110 044

SAGE Publications Asia-Pacific Pte Ltd
3 Church Street
#10-04 Samsung Hub
Singapore 049483

Editor: Becky Taylor
Associate editor: Emma Milman
Production editor: Katie Forsythe
Copyeditor: Solveig Gardner Servian
Proofreader: Tom Bedford
Marketing manager: Camille Richmond
Cover design: Wendy Scott
Typeset by: C&M Digitals (P) Ltd, Chennai, India
Printed and bound by CPI Group (UK) Ltd,
Croydon, CR0 4YY

Editorial arrangement and Chapters 1, 2, 5, 6, 7, 8, 9, 10 ©
Michelle Brown 2016
Chapters 3 and 4 © Michelle Brown and Kersten Hardy 2016
Chapter 11 © Martin Brock and Michelle Brown 2016

First published 2016

**Library of Congress Control Number: 2015949240**

**British Library Cataloguing in Publication data**

A catalogue record for this book is available from
the British Library

ISBN 978-1-4462-9568-7
ISBN 978-1-4462-9569-4 (pbk)

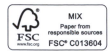

MIX
Paper from
responsible sources
FSC
www.fsc.org    FSC® C013604

At SAGE we take sustainability seriously. Most of our products are printed in the UK using FSC papers and boards.
When we print overseas we ensure sustainable papers are used as measured by the Egmont grading system.
We undertake an annual audit to monitor our sustainability.

# Contents

# About the editor and contributors

**Michelle Brown** currently works at the University of Derby as a senior lecturer. Her clinical practice has incorporated oncology and palliative care nursing. Before qualifying, she knew that caring for people with a life-limiting illness was what she wanted. Once qualified, after a small number of posts, she managed to attain a post on a gastrointestinal surgery ward. This often involved helping, supporting and caring for patients with a cancer diagnosis pre- and post-operatively. From there she spent a number of years in urology oncology research then working as a clinical nurse specialist. It was whilst working in this role, caring for individuals with a life-limiting illness, breaking bad news and liaising with palliative care specialists that she realised that she needed to be working in the palliative care field. She was fortunate enough to be able to undertake a Master's degree in palliative care in the Trent Palliative Care Centre with the University of Sheffield. She felt inspired and applied for a hospice post. Although she was employed by the hospice, her role involved working in an acute Trust. This was demanding but rewarding. Referrals included cancer and non-cancer diagnoses but in addition there were a number of patients who were cancer survivors.

Unfortunately there was little time for teaching other than ad-hoc, micro-teaching with nursing and medical staff. Michelle really wanted to improve the care that patients and their loved ones received, therefore, she made a very difficult decision and applied for a lecturing post. This post has given Michelle the flexibility to write, maintain clinical practice when she can, but also to try to inspire others as she had been during her Master's degree. Michelle sincerely hopes that this book will help you understand her passion but also help you to develop your skills and knowledge in order to provide high-quality palliative and end of life care to those with a life-limiting illness.

**Martin Brock** (MSc) is a Registered Mental Health Nurse and an accredited Cognitive Behavioural Psychotherapist with some 34 years clinical experience. He has trained clinically in Acceptance and Commitment Therapy, Compassion Focused Therapy and Mindfulness Based Cognitive Therapy and has a thriving private practice.

Martin is a fellow of the Higher Education Academy in the UK and a Senior Lecturer at the University of Derby with a specific focus on teaching and researching compassionate practice in healthcare.

**Kersten Hardy** works in the community as a Band 5 Staff Nurse, a post she has held since June 2014. Within this role, Kersten cares for many vulnerable and dependent patients in their own home that need the input of a registered nurse, but do not require admission into hospital. This role puts her in contact with many different health needs and disciplines, predominantly, and most importantly, patients who require palliative/supportive and end of life care, but wish to stay in their home environment.

Kersten found palliative care almost by accident, starting work as a care assistant at a local hospice in 2001. In the first few weeks she feared this environment was not somewhere she could work and began to look for another job, but seven years later she was still working at the hospice and was extremely passionate about the care and service delivered to all that needed help. Kersten was encouraged and supported to train as a nurse, which she did, qualifying in May 2010 with an Advanced Diploma in Nursing Studies from the University of Derby.

In September 2011 Kersten was lucky enough to secure a job back at her local hospice where it all began. She continued in her role but the more she thought about the role the more she wanted to focus on delivering palliative care to patients in their own homes, so she searched for an area of work that would enable her to do this, which brings her to where she is today. Kersten continued her education and topped her ADNS into a BSc, inclusive of a palliative care module and focusing her dissertation on 'delirium at the end of life', obtaining a first class honours.

In the 14 years that Kersten has been in the palliative care environment she has seen many changes in the treatment and management of many life-limiting illnesses, as well as the positive impact of good palliative/supportive care and the areas that still need a lot of input. She hopes, in the future, to be able to contribute to the fast moving developments, but in the interim she will continue to do what she can, where she can, to ensure good patient care and will work towards starting and completing a MSc in Supportive and Palliative Care.

# About this book

I would like to inspire and help all those interested in delivering the best care: this book encourages reflection around your own experiences but also introduces a number of case studies to help make sense of the theories, policies and guidance which support palliative and end of life care delivery. An international perspective is also provided, as the evidence suggests that there are issues surrounding care at the end of life globally. This book is suitable for undergraduate students and for postgraduate healthcare professionals who want a practical book to help them make sense of caring for an individual with a life-limiting illness.

Chapter 1 examines palliative care from a historical perspective, and then goes on to look at the present and what the future holds. It examines some of the fundamental issues in palliative and supportive care.

Chapter 2 discusses care and compassion for those with a life-limiting illness and addresses the needs of those with cancer and non-cancer diagnoses. It addresses quality in palliative care and how we can achieve it using a team approach.

Chapter 3 examines holistic assessment and why this is paramount when caring for an individual with a life-limiting illness. A number of assessment tools are considered, as is the contribution that the interprofessional team can make to holistic care.

Chapter 4 looks at planning care. It covers the why, what and how of care planning. Care planning will be discussed in general followed by an examination of care planning for those with a life-limiting illness and through to end of life care.

Chapter 5 addresses carers' needs. Caring has a significant impact on carers' health and this will be discussed within the chapter. Suggestions will be made regarding how we can help carers continue to provide care.

Chapter 6 discusses the interprofessional approach to care. It will explore team roles and how they may contribute to the delivery of high-quality palliative and end of life care. Some challenges to effective interprofessional working are also addressed.

Chapter 7 examines communication in palliative and end of life care. It discusses the importance of communication when an individual is faced with their own mortality. The evidence surrounding what people want from healthcare professionals at the end of life will also be explored.

Chapter 8 discusses some key ethical issues in palliative and end of life care. The role ethics plays in helping to make difficult decisions will be explored. A number of legal concerns will also be examined, e.g. the Mental Capacity Act.

Chapter 9 addresses end of life care. Philosophies underpinning end of life care as well as some of the difficulties and challenges that face healthcare professionals, patients and carers when an individual is approaching end of life.

Chapter 10 looks at death and dying. Establishing when time is short for your patient is often one of the key issues in end of life care. This will be addressed and the chapter explores a 'good death'.

Chapter 11, the final chapter, is a restorative chapter. It is there to ensure you have the ability to care for yourself. Palliative and end of life care can be challenging. What we need to ensure is that we have the ability to maintain a compassionate approach and to achieve this we need to be compassionate to ourselves. This chapter contains some useful advice and help. It suggests exercises to do in order to maintain your self-compassion and prevent the potential for emotional fatigue.

## How to use this book

This book can be read from cover to cover during your studies, and you can also dip in and out of it once you qualify to help you reflect on particular issues or concerns you may come across during practice. There are useful reflective case studies to help make sense of the discussion and add some reality to the text. There is also some recommended reading which supports each specific chapter.

The philosophy of this book is that it should be easy to read and engaging, but also should inspire you to make a difference by delivering high-quality palliative and end of life care with a little more confidence.

And finally! High-quality palliative care is not just about doing your job well and making sure people are safe, it is about life and death. The experience touches a huge number of people's lives. You can have a positive effect on not only the patients' lives but also that of their carers' and loved ones, and that memory will live on.

Michelle Brown

# 1

# Palliative care past, present and the future

This chapter will explore:

- the philosophy underpinning palliative care
- the journey that palliative care provision has taken and where we are now
- the tools available to help care for those with a life-limiting condition
- the palliative care needs of patients with a life-limiting illness including those with a non-cancer diagnosis.

## Reflection points

Start by thinking about these reflection points:

- What is palliative care?
- Who can access palliative care services?
- Who delivers palliative care?

## Palliative care and its goals

> You matter because you are you. You matter to the last moment of your life, and we will do all we can not only to help you die peacefully, but to live until you die. (Saunders 1976: 1003–4)

As nurses, we work with patients in order to promote and achieve individualised care. This is because we recognise that a patient is not just a set of physical symptoms or a diagnosis, they are also a physical being with psychological, social, spiritual and emotional needs. Identifying what is important to each individual patient helps us to prioritise their care needs and helps to ensure that we support them and create the optimum quality of life for that individual right up until their death. The concept of a 'good death' is what we all strive for as professionals, and therefore assisting a patient in achieving that should be our ultimate goal and indeed our responsibility.

## Palliative care from the beginning

The hospice movement developed its impetus in the 1960s and 1970s. One of the key drivers in initiating this dynamic change was Cicely Saunders (later to become Dame). She generated a new vision surrounding caring for those at the end of life. It was one which incorporated a holistic view of the patient rather than seeing them as a set of physical symptoms. She achieved this vision by engaging and listening to the individuals in her care and noted that they were experiencing more than just physical symptoms, believing that these physical symptoms had psychological, emotional, social and spiritual components.

The goal of palliative care is to achieve the best possible quality of life for patients and their families (World Health Organization (WHO) 1990). 'Palliatus' is a Latin term meaning 'to cloak or conceal', therefore palliative care involves utilising comprehensive holistic assessments and adopting appropriate treatment strategies in order to improve quality of life for those with a life-limiting illness (Claxton-Oldfield et al. 2004). There are a number of ways that we can treat a patient with a life-limiting illness; for example, medical palliation is the active relief of a symptom or a problem which does not necessarily affect lifespan. Palliative care does not simply involve the administration of a cocktail of drugs (pharmacotherapy), but also involves a multitude of interventions in order to help, support and care for those patients and their carer and/or relative. Symptoms may be multidimensional, meaning they do not only derive from a physical problem. An example could be a patient who has heart failure and feels that she is dying. She may have other psychological issues as her husband died in a distressed state from heart failure five years before. In addition, she may have severed contact with friends because she may not want to burden them or feel like socialising due to her current state of health. This would mean that she has emotional, psychological and social issues which may be exacerbating her condition, so dealing with only physical symptoms would not address the whole problem. Holistic assessment is the key to addressing any issues or aspects that may be contributing to the patient's diminished quality of life.

## Palliative care: the present

There have been dynamic changes in palliative care provision within the UK to improve palliative and supportive care provision. These changes have been driven by research, recommendations, strategies and policy. The pivotal points include the introduction of the Department of Health's *End of Life Care Strategy* (DH 2008) and the introduction of the Gold Standards Framework (Thomas 2003; National Health Service (NHS), Royal College of General Practitioners 2006). These frameworks alongside many other publications suggest standards of care that should be employed when caring for a patient and their family as they approach the end of life, including the opportunity to decide where and how they would like their care to be delivered (NHS 2014). The preferred place of care (PPC) allows a person to be cared for in an environment of their choice, which may be home, hospital nursing home or hospice (see Chapters 9 and 10 for further discussion). The National Institute for Health and Care Excellence (NICE) (2011b) stated that we should optimise the amount of time people spend in their PPC during the last year of life. To enable this to happen, coordinated, high-quality care is needed so that the individual feels confident that the care delivered is meeting their needs and that they are comfortable in the PPC. NICE have, in addition, produced standards to aid high quality end of life care which include: 'improving supportive and palliative care for adults with cancer' (2004); lung cancer guidance (2011a); standards for care at the end of life (2011b); and the use of opioids in end of life care (2012). Currently further guidance is being compiled including care of the dying adult (NICE 2015a, b, c), an update surrounding improving supportive and palliative care adults, due in 2018 and guidance for end of life care for infants, children and young people in 2016. In addition, organisations have been developed and work in collaboration with the National Health Service and Department of Health, such as the National Coalition for Hospice and Palliative Care (NCHPC), National End of Life Care Intelligence Network (NEoLCIN) and The Marie Curie Palliative Care Institute Liverpool (MCPCIL), to drive the quality of services in palliative and end of life care. The guidance available embraces common themes, which include the recognition that clear communication between all the members of the multidisciplinary team and the patient is paramount. In addition, education and support for staff caring for individuals with a life-limiting illness and the need to ensure that patients are central to all decision making using enhanced and effective communication skills are vital.

The issues are that worldwide, there is a lack of education and knowledge in those caring for people in the palliative phase of illness, yet the need for palliative and end of life care is significant and increasing (WHO 2014). Over 19 million people worldwide need palliative care, with 69 per cent of those being over the age of 65 (WHO 2014), so this sets an enormous task as health and social care professionals need to have some understanding about how to care for these individuals using the philosophies and standards suggested (see Figure 1.1).

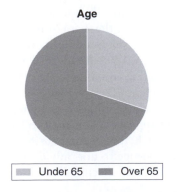

**Figure 1.1** Age of people requiring palliative care (WHO 2014)

This cannot be achieved without addressing people's educational needs and supporting them in achieving the competence and confidence required to provide the high-quality palliative and end of life care everyone deserves. There are inherent difficulties in ensuring that patients receive high-quality palliative and end of life care, no matter where the patient is. In acute hospitals this may be challenging due to the environment itself (e.g. lack of privacy, lack of peace and quiet if they require it). There are challenges for staff regarding the need to spend time with those nearing end of life and to give them the care they need whilst at the same time attending to patients with acute ill health who need urgent attention. Trying to meet everyone's needs is a dilemma in itself.

## Palliative care models and tools

Tools have been designed and introduced to assist in the delivery of integrated high-quality end of life care no matter where it is delivered. The Liverpool Care Pathway introduced in the 1990s was adopted as best practice by NICE and the DH (Ellershaw et al. 1997; DH 2008; NICE 2004). This was an integrated care pathway and was developed as a tool to help those caring for patients in the last weeks or days of life. Its philosophy emanated from the hospice approach to care at the end of life, which is regarded as 'gold standard'. As very few people at the end of life have access to the hospice environment the tool was developed to aid equity in end of life care (Kinder and Ellershaw 2003; National Audit Office (NAO) 2008). The aim was to prompt healthcare professionals to consider communication needs and signpost staff and patients through the last days of life in order to ensure that a good standard of care was achieved. Although this was the aim, The Marie Curie Palliative Care Institute Liverpool and the Royal College of Physicians conducted an investigation which focused on the care received by patients who had been placed on the pathway (2007): the final report suggested that the physical domains of care demonstrated good compliance with the pathway but the spiritual and psychological domains demonstrated minimal compliance, with communication between the healthcare professional and patient once again being poor. The Liverpool Care Pathway received negative attention, although the premise regarding its ethos is widely accepted as positive. There may be numerous reasons why this tool created such public and professional outcry; these could include misunderstanding through lack of knowledge and education surrounding its implementation amongst healthcare professionals. The Liverpool Care Pathway was phased out, and in its place came further guidance surrounding end of life care planning in the publication *More Care, Less Pathway* (Independent Review Panel of the Liverpool Care Pathway 2013). This recommends that end of life care plans which are unique and individualised should be the preferred approach. One may still argue that the implementation of this requires a robust approach, that ensures staff have undergone adequate training and possess sufficient knowledge to not only develop the plan, but also have the ability and communication skills to discuss choices at the end of life. In addition, comprehensive, disease-specific guides will be introduced as well as manuals which reflect the principles of good palliative care. If this strategy for caring at the end of life is accomplished, then a calm and informed approach may be adopted for those approaching the end of life rather than the frenetic, ill-informed management which often results in a less than adequate experience for all concerned and we must remember that this is not something we can go back and change.

## The palliative care approach

Internationally, palliative care has been provided for hundreds of years, but today's philosophy promotes a patient-centred approach which should be delivered by knowledgeable and skilled healthcare professionals in order to ensure that high-standard, evidence-based care is achieved. Palliative care involves treating symptoms to maximise quality of life, it should not attempt to postpone or hasten death (WHO 1990). It perceives death and dying as normal processes rather than failures, and affirms life and living but not at the expense of quality of life (National Council for Hospice and Palliative Care Services 2001). The staff delivering palliative care may be diverse, for example, dietician, physiotherapist, social worker. One recommendation within the NICE standards (2004) and the *End of Life Care Strategy* (DH 2008) is that a professional with specialist expertise in the field of practice should be employed to help support the patient throughout their journey and refer to other disciplines as necessary. This may not be accessible to all, and Skilbeck and Payne (2005) suggest that for patients requiring a 'palliative care approach', this can be delivered by staff who have been supported and educated appropriately, but that there may be patients who have complex symptoms or a range of needs which require more specialist input, and it is this specialist input that NICE (2004, 2011b) and the Department of Health (2008) are suggesting must meet these needs. This should be available for patients with cancer and non-cancer diagnoses. The difficulty is knowing whether or not all of this can be achieved. Being able to coordinate care delivery in negotiation with the patient is a privileged role but one that requires a sound evidence base, continuous professional development and higher-level understanding. NICE (2004) suggested that this member of staff should undergo communication assessment in order to ensure that they have the necessary enhanced skills to support the patient and their relatives through a difficult journey. This member of staff could not see all the patients in that specialist area, therefore organisations need to invest in their staff to ensure that those involved in caring for patients at the end of life have an adequate skill and knowledge base to provide effective care that is of a good standard.

Many of the frameworks elaborate and suggest standards surrounding end of life care (DH 2008; NICE 2004, 2011b). Palliative care however, does not only involve care at the end of life. It is paramount that definitions are clearly explained. Palliative care entails care delivered by a diverse range of professionals using a holistic approach to a patient whose illness is deemed incurable. The aim should be to improve a patient's quality of life and that of their carer (WHO 2002). End of life or terminal care should focus on the few last weeks, days or hours of a patient's life, where the focus becomes patient comfort, and a great deal of preparation surrounding needs and wishes at the end of life are essential. Advance directives are a means of establishing patient's wishes as they approach the end of life (see Chapter 8 for further discussion). They need to be clear and can be implemented if a patient no longer has the capacity to make decisions about treatments or interventions (see Chapter 8). The National Council for Palliative Care (2014) suggest that individuals approaching the end of life have the right to the highest-quality care and support, wherever they live and whatever their condition, and that those with a life-limiting condition other than cancer should have the same equity of access to high-quality palliative care as those with a cancer diagnosis. This is not a new idea but it has taken some time to address this challenge. There does now appear to be a greater equity in access, but with this comes significant challenges in educating those healthcare professionals who are to deliver this high standard of palliative care.

Let us consider some definitions synonymous with a patient's journey through palliative care to end of life.

---

### 👥 Case scenario: George

George was 55 when he was diagnosed with prostate cancer. He underwent radical (potentially curative) surgery to remove the cancer. At this point he was in the curative phase of his illness. Eighteen months after his surgery the cancer had returned and it was deemed incurable but treatable with hormonal manipulation therapy. This would not cure him but would keep the disease stable for a period of time. One could then suggest that George is in the palliative phase of illness, and this may be a protracted period where he has symptoms relating to his disease or treatments and these may be distressing. Intervention revolves around treating any symptoms in order to maximise his quality of life.

George continues on this treatment for five years, but at his follow-up his blood tests suggest his cancer is now growing again and he complains of back pain. On investigation George was informed that his cancer was now advancing and treatments would involve trying to slow the progression rate and treat his symptoms. This could be radiotherapy (X-ray treatment) to his back alongside pain relief together with an attempt at further drug management for the cancer.

George deteriorates further over the next six months and it is clear that his disease is extremely advanced. He is suffering with severe pain, nausea, constipation, fatigue and anorexia. He needs regular rest and his blood tests suggest that the cancer has spread beyond the prostate and bones. The prognosis is poor, with an advancing decline evident. George is now entering the terminal phase of his illness with the expectation that time may be quite short. Care at this point should focus on George's comfort, using medication and complementary therapies to promote his dignity in the last days of life.

## Reflection points

- Can you see how George's illness progresses?
- What physical, psychological, spiritual and social needs do you think George will have as his illness progresses?

An environment of calm where loved ones can be near and where everyone feels supported is paramount to aid a dignified and peaceful death. This exemplar is quite clear when dealing with a patient with cancer but can become extremely difficult when a patient has a non-cancer diagnosis, as the unpredictability regarding the course of the condition can make planning for a peaceful and dignified death a challenge. Decisions may have to be made swiftly, and lack of recognition that a patient is entering the terminal phase of illness is a common issue. The nature of the diseases (e.g. multiple sclerosis, COPD, heart failure etc.) all entail periods of exacerbations and remissions and the challenge is to identify when an exacerbation precedes the terminal phase of illness. There may also be difficulty in initiating a discussion surrounding wishes for end of life care, as deterioration may have no definite or significant time-point, which may be more apparent for those with a cancer diagnosis. Access to specialist services may be hindered by the time constraints involved in recognising that a patient is approaching the end of life.

Care delivery should be underpinned with a holistic philosophy: caring for the whole person and ensuring that their anxieties and fears are given just as much attention as more physical symptoms such as vomiting or constipation. The following chapters in this book should help you to identify George's needs as his illness progresses.

## Palliative care needs internationally

Internationally there are many commonalities in the requirements that patients and relatives have at the end of life. Dy et al. (2007) conducted a systematic review focusing on satisfaction with care at the end of life. Satisfaction was an important aspect regarding perceived quality of care, and the key themes emerging from this review were the accessibility of end of life care services and the coordination of those services (see Figure 1.2). Although the review presented an international perspective one may argue that this is a generalisable view of many who are receiving palliative and end of life care. In addition to these requirements, symptom management, comfort in death, communication and education as well as spiritual and emotional support were all prerequisites to a 'good death'.

These themes were not disease specific but common amongst the numerous conditions. The aims for palliative care within the UK concur with the perceptions from these patients and relatives within the studies examined in the review. High-quality

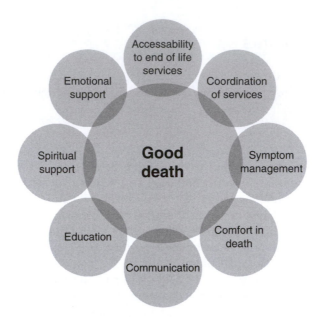

**Figure 1.2**    Factors influencing a 'good death' (Dy et al. 2007)

palliative care is not a luxury but should be seen as a significant international pub-lic health concern (WHO 2014; Foley 2003). What appears to be the undeniable requirement in achieving these goals for patients and their carers is knowledgeable, compassionate staff. Improving satisfaction is a means of improving the experience of those approaching the end of life (Dy et al. 2007).

## Supportive and palliative care

Palliative care has undergone continued changes, with the acknowledgement that terming the specialist field 'supportive and palliative care' may be a more accurate representation of the interventions it employs. Patients and their relatives may be suffering physically, psychologically, emotionally, socially and/or spiritually at diag-nosis. Specialist teams may be competent in managing a range of issues presented, but in addition the palliative care team may be able to offer a different but comple-mentary dimension to the disease-specific specialist team. One may argue that introducing palliative care at an earlier stage may also dispel the myths and image of palliative care specialism as end of life care, therefore encouraging people who are struggling with symptoms to be less apprehensive and fearful of specialist pal-liative care involvement or referral should it be needed.

Within the UK, Palliative care as a specialist field of practice has been a relatively recent provision. The teamwork and collaborative approach involved in helping and caring for patients and their loved ones is essential in ensuring that a seam-less multidimensional approach is adopted. Patients often have complex needs which incorporate more than just physical symptoms or in some cases may not even include any physical presentation. In a study by Skilbeck et al. (2002), 57 per cent of the 814 referrals the palliative care team received were for emotional support. This suggests that a large number of patients are struggling psychologically and emotionally with their diagnosis. Despite this research preceding many of the policies and standards introduced over the last decade which aimed to address these concerns, psychosocial issues and communication skills remain unacknowledged and unresolved for many patients (Healthcare Commission 2008). The holistic assessment should be fundamental and initiate caring for the whole person rather than the physical symptoms alone. (See Chapter 3 for further discussion.)

## Long-term conditions and palliative care

Traditionally those accessing palliative care services were patients with a cancer diagnosis, but there has been a growing recognition that this has provided an inequitable service for those with a non-cancer diagnosis but still suffering a life-limiting illness. Skilbeck and Payne (2005) argue that palliative and end of life care for those with a chronic long-term condition (LTC) remains fragmented, with poor symptom control and limited access to specialist palliative care services. This demonstrates that significant inequities continue to exist, and one may argue that effective symptom control and support will be needed no matter what the diagnosis. In Skilbeck et al.'s study (2002), although a little dated, they found that when examining the referrals made to the specialist palliative care team over a 1-year duration, only 3 per cent of the referrals had a non-cancer diagnosis. When a patient is facing a life-limiting condition they have a number of needs, including dealing with anxieties about their own mortality and death. In a United States (US) study, Tilden and Thompson (1999) identified that Americans fear how they die more than the death itself because of the advancements in medical technology which may lead to extensive, aggressive medical management of those with a life-limiting illness. This may be exacerbated when there are difficulties in identifying the end of life for those with a non-malignant disease. Therefore admissions to critical care areas when a patient is in fact nearing the end of life may be difficult to manage for the staff, patients and relatives due to conflicts regarding what is in the best interest of the patient and the high expectations of the patient and relatives. These dilemmas were identified in Beckstrand et al.'s (2006) multicentre study examining nurses' perceptions of a 'good death' in critical care. The environment where end of life care is delivered can have an impact on the perceived quality of that care. The intensive care unit can often witness a degree of conflict, and this was evident in the participants' responses. These were extremely varied and the dominant themes are shown in Figure 1.3.

Most reported lack of knowledge when it came to optimising a good death as they felt that both their pre-registration and post-registration education did not prepare them adequately. What is apparent from this study is that end of life care creates a great deal of anxiety for the staff attempting to provide high-quality care and a good death. Lack of preparation for dealing with these end of life issues appears to affect

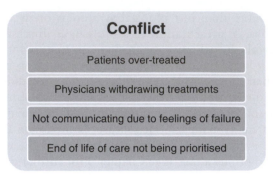

**Figure 1.3**   Influences on conflict (Beckstrand et al. 2006)

the care given. Education and training appear to be clear key messages from this study, and it is likely that this is transferable to other intensive treatment units as well as to many other healthcare settings and specialist areas. These issues will be examined in more detail throughout this book.

The profile of those needing palliative care is shifting due to the changing nature of health needs. As the number of adults over the age of 65 increases, there is a rising incidence of diagnosed LTCs. More people die due to LTCs than cancer (Office for National Statistics 2008). It is estimated that 70 per cent of the National Health Service budget is spent on treating patients for their LTC (Joint Commission Panel for Mental Health (JCPMH) 2012). These LTC's can present with a multitude of difficulties for the patient and their carer, as generally the older person may present with multiple problems incorporating other co-morbidities which may make the management and care more demanding and complex (Ridgeway 2011). The JCPMH (2012) identify that LTCs are generally associated with more mental health issues, therefore they require comprehensive, holistic assessment and treatment in order to meet and address their needs. Myriad psychosocial, physical and spiritual issues may not only have a negative impact on the quality of life of the patients, but may once again present numerous issues for the carer. One example would be the incidence of low mood. Those with a LTC may be two or three times more likely to suffer significant depression (Haddad 2010). This may have an impact on their desire to seek interventions and could affect them in the physical, spiritual and social domains, restricting their desire to socialise and induce feelings of worthlessness. The incidence of depression and impact a diagnosis of chronic obstructive pulmonary disease (COPD) has on individuals equates to the significant symptom presentations a patient with lung cancer may have. The difference is that the patient with COPD may experience a protracted illness where quality of life gradually diminishes (Shuttleworth 2005). Ahmedzai (2003) examined the burden of progressive non-malignant lung disease in some depth and identified that patients require supportive care throughout their journey and that holistic assessment should be the cornerstone of nursing care delivery in order to maximise quality of life. The Royal College of Psychiatrists (2009) identified that one-quarter of the patients in their studies with physical illness developed a mental illness. It was felt that trying to live with the burden of disease and for those with a potential life-threatening disorder, this may be more pronounced. These issues will have a significant impact on our practice as we may find ourselves providing significantly more palliative and terminal-phase care than ever before as demand increases from those suffering with LTCs. Providing palliative care demands a certain level of self-awareness and clarity regarding our own beliefs, values and knowledge (Baldwin 2011). Dealing with significant distress can have a long-term impact on our own wellbeing as we too experience grief and bereavement, therefore the last chapter of this book will examine ways of helping ourselves and strategies we can use to identify our own distress and burden.

Within the UK there is now recognition that any patient with a life-limiting illness should have access to any service or support they require when they need it no matter what their diagnosis. This has ensured a fair and just provision for all who are suffering. This applies not only to justice for those with any illness, but includes justice for all individuals who may be marginalised (e.g. the elderly, those in prison, travellers and culturally diverse groups). Although these groups have been traditionally 'hard to reach' and may find accessing services difficult, there is a growing need to restructure service provision in order to meet their needs. To reiterate however, access may be available but this relies on the recognition that the patient is at the point where they need palliative or end of life care.

## Communication

The Department of Health (2008) and NICE (2004) introduced strategies and guidance in order to promote access for all and suggested a clear minimum standard of care. They recommended improvements in the communication strategies currently employed and that more collaborative working within the multidisciplinary team should be encompassed in order to facilitate high-quality end of life care. Effective communication strategies are needed to ensure that this comprehensive approach is seamlessly channelled to all those aiming to achieve similar goals for the benefit of the patient and their relatives. Those requiring palliative care input may have complex needs; consequently, health and social care providers need to meet these multiple aspects of patient need. Patient-centred care, inclusivity in decision making and empowerment incorporate the essence of palliative care delivery. Effective communication throughout the patient's journey is fundamental in delivering these goals (DH 2008).

## Knowledge

Palliative care is not only delivered by palliative care teams. In the Royal Liverpool Hospital the Palliative Care Team had contact with only 15 per cent of those who died in the hospital (Kinder and Ellershaw 2003). When one considers that 65 per cent of deaths occur in hospital, there are a significant number of patients who die in hospital under the care of the nursing staff on the ward. What this shows is that ward staff are often providing palliative care to a large patient group, so it is vital that they are knowledgeable and properly equipped to care for these patients. In the community setting, including nursing homes, many district nursing teams and nursing home staff provide excellent nursing care to those with a life-limiting illness. The Parliamentary and Health Service Ombudsman (2015) stated that individuals should have access to specialist palliative care services no matter what diagnosis, when they need it, but also that those providing care at the end of life should be knowledgeable and confident enough to ensure that symptoms are addressed and managed to prevent suffering. This may mean that specialist palliative care teams take on a more educational role and then intervene when a patient is suffering due to very complex problems.

The Department of Health in 2008 had identified similar issues, suggesting that sub-optimal end of life care was prolific throughout National Health Service provision and attributed this to poor knowledge base and lack of educational opportunities. As a consequence investment in staff was viewed as paramount to ensure that those vulnerable groups with life-limiting illness could be assured a more proactive approach to their care that was evidence based and delivered by knowledgeable practitioners. What one should acknowledge is that support and education for these staff needs to be on-going. Nurses have a responsibility to ensure the patient and their carers receive high-quality, evidence-based care (Nursing and Midwifery Council (NMC) 2015).

## Conclusion

The need to provide equity in palliative care delivery is not only a UK goal but has been recognised as a significant issue globally. As far back as 2005, the 2nd Global Summit of National Hospice and Palliative Care Associations (PCA) identified the need to ensure that equity in access was paramount no matter what race, gender, diagnosis, sexual orientation, culture or religion. As a result the Korean Declaration on Hospice and Palliative Care was developed (International Association for Hospice and Palliative Care 2005). Within the UK, the end of life care strategy demanded that equity is a human right and therefore access to high-quality palliative and end of life care should be facilitated and provided to all who need it (DH 2008). Ensuring that we have adequate training and education both pre-registration and post-registration is the nurse's responsibility (NMC 2010). The delivery of services should be compassion-led, creating a therapeutic relationship with our patients, carers and service users. One outcome of the Francis report, *Compassion in Practice* (DH 2012), supported the concept of 'the 6 Cs' (care, compassion, competence, courage, communication and commitment). Additional guidance was launched, which included ensuring shared decision making and communication with those in our care and collaboration with others. These are pertinent goals when one considers that living well and dying well are the fundamental needs of patients approaching the end of life. We can deliver the high-quality care needed to ensure dignity and serenity as the end of life approaches.

## Reflection points

- Has your understanding changed?
- What is your understanding of palliative care now?
- Consider this scenario and complete the reflection points at the end.

### 📠 Case scenario: Beryl

Beryl is 47 and she has been referred to the district nursing team having received a diagnosis of lung cancer. She felt overwhelmed when the news came. There were a number of professionals in the room but she cannot recall much of what was said. Her first thought when she was told was her children and what would happen to them. The only recollection was that it wasn't curable and she was awaiting palliative treatment which would help her symptoms.

She is a single parent and works full time as a secretary. She has two children, Thomas 14 and Jessica 9. Her husband died six years earlier following a road traffic accident. The children have accepted the loss of their father although it was extremely difficult for a number of months afterwards. Beryl has some contact with her mother but she lives 240 miles away and therefore contact is generally via the telephone. She has friends but does not really socialise as she prefers to spend her time with the children.

Beryl has a mortgage on her house, she struggles but manages to have a reasonable standard of living.

The diagnosis has been a great shock and she is struggling to think about what is going to happen and make plans for the future. She does feel that she needs some help with this as she does not seem to be able to think straight.

Currently her symptoms include pain, nausea, insomnia, breathlessness and fatigue. The distressing symptom is her fatigue because she feels she needs to be as active as possible for the sake of the children.

## Reflection points

- What is important when you discuss Beryl's care with her?
- List the health and social care professionals that may help to support and care for Beryl.
- How can we help the children?
- Are there any agencies that may be able to help Beryl?
- Think about why you have made your decisions.
- Why would a holistic assessment be important here?

## Suggested reading

Department of Health (2008) *End of Life Care Strategy*. London: DH.
Department of Health (2012) *Compassion in Practice*. London: DH.

## Useful websites

National Council for Palliative Care: www.ncpc.org.uk

# References

Ahmedzai, S.H. (2003) *Terminal Care in Non-malignant, End-stage Disease: How Can We Improve It?* Presentation at the Royal College of Physicians of Edinburgh. Edinburgh: RCPE.

Baldwin, M. (2011) 'Hospice movement and evolution of palliative care', in M. Baldwin and J. Woodhouse (eds), *Key Concepts in Palliative Care*. London: Sage, pp. 92–6.

Beckstrand, R.L., Clark Callister, L. and Kirchhoff, K.T. (2006) 'Providing a "good death": Critical care nurses' suggestions for improving end of life care', *American Journal of Critical Care*, 15: 38–45.

Claxton-Oldfield, S., Claxton-Oldfield, J. and Rishchynski, G. (2004) 'Understanding of the term "palliative care": A Canadian survey', *American Journal of Hospital and Palliative Medicine*, 21(2): 105–10.

Department of Health (2008) *End of Life Care Strategy*. London: DH.

Department of Health (2012) *Compassion in Practice*. London: DH.

Dy, S.M., Shugarman, L.R., Lorenz, K.A., Mularski, R.A., Lynn, J., for the RAND-Southern California Evidence-Based Practice Centre (2007) 'A systematic review of satisfaction with care at the end of life', *Journal of the American Geriatric Society*, 56: 1.

Ellershaw, J., Murphy, D., Shea, T., Foster, A. and Overill, S. (1997) 'Developing an integrated care pathway for the dying patient', *European Journal of Palliative Care*, 4: 203–8.

Foley, K. (2003) 'How much palliative care do we need?', *European Journal of Palliative Care*, 10: 5–7.

Haddad, M. (2010) 'Caring for patients with long-term conditions and depression', *Nursing Standard*, 24(24): 40–9.

Healthcare Commission (2008) *Spotlight on Complaints: A Report on Second Stage Complaints about the NHS in England*. London: Healthcare Commission.

Independent Review of the Liverpool Care Pathway Panel (2013) *More Care, Less Pathway: A Review of the Liverpool Care Pathway*. London: Crown Copyright.

International Association for Hospice and Palliative Care (2005) 2nd Global Summit of National Hospice and Palliative Care Associations, March, Korea. Accessed at: www.hospicecare.com/newsletter2005/apr05/global.html (accessed 15.7.2015).

Joint Commission Panel for Mental Health (2012) *Guidance for Commissioners of Liaison Mental Health Services to Acute Hospitals. Volume II: Practical Mental Health Commissioning*. London: JCPMH.

Kinder, C. and Ellershaw, J. (2003) 'How to use Liverpool Care Pathway for the dying patient', in C. Kinder and J. Ellershaw (eds), *Care of the Dying, a Pathway to Excellence*. Oxford: Oxford University Press, pp. 11–41.

Marie Curie Palliative Care Institute Liverpool and the Royal College of Physicians (2007) *National Care of the Dying Audit – Hospitals (2007)*. London: RCP.

National Audit Office (2008) *End of Life Care*. London: The Stationery Office.

National Council for Hospice and Palliative Care Services (2001) *Raising Awareness of Death, Dying and Bereavement*. London: NCPC. Available at: www.dyingmatters.org/page/what-palliative-care (accessed 22.4.13).

National Council for Palliative Care (2014) *About NCPC*. London: NCPC. Available at: www.ncpc.org.uk (accessed 4.6.15).

National Health Service (2014) *Actions for End of Life Care 2014–2016*. London: NHS.

National Health Service, Gold Standards Framework, Royal College of General Practitioners (2006) *Prognostic Indicator Guidance: to Aid Identification of Adult Patients with Advanced Disease, in the Last Months/Year of Life, Who Are in Need of Supportive and*

*Palliative Care*. Birmingham: Gold Standards Framework National Team, Birmingham. Available at: www.goldstandardsframework.nhs.uk/content/gp_contract/Prognostic%20 Indicators%20Guidance20Paper%20v%2025 (accessed 25.11.13).

National Institute for Health and Care Excellence (2004) *Guidance on Cancer Services: Improving Supportive and Palliative Care for Adults with Cancer: The Manual*. London: NICE.

National Institute for Health and Care Excellence (2011a) *CG121 Lung Cancer: The Diagnosis and Treatment of Lung Cancer*. London: NICE.

National Institute for Health and Care Excellence (2011b) *Quality Standard for End of Life Care for Adults*. London: NICE.

National Institute for Health and Care Excellence (2012) *Opioids in Palliative Care: Safe and Effective Prescribing of Strong Opioids for Pain in Palliative Care of Adults*. London: NICE.

National Institute for Health and Care Excellence (2015a) *Care of the Dying Adult: Guidance In Progress*. London: NICE. Available at: www.nice.org.uk/guidance/indevelopment/gid-cgwave0694 (accessed 20 August 2015).

National Institute for Health and Care Excellence (2015b) *End of Life Care For Infants, Children and Young People*. London: NICE. Available at: www.nice.org.uk/guidance/indevelopment/gid-cgwave0730 (accessed 20 August 2015).

National Institute for Health and Care Excellence (2015c) *Improving Supportive and Palliative Care in Adults*. England, NICE. Available at: www.nice.org.uk/guidance/indevelopment/gid-cgwave0799 (accessed 20 August 2015).

Nursing and Midwifery Council (2010) *Standards for Pre-registration Education*. London: NMC.

Nursing and Midwifery Council (2015) *The Code: Professional Standards of Practice and Behaviour for Nurses and Midwives*. London: NMC.

Office for National Statistics (2008) *Mortality Statistics*. London: ONS.

Parliamentary and Health Service Ombudsman (2015) *Dying without Dignity. Investigations by the Parliamentary and Health Service Ombudsman into Complaints about End of Life Care*. London: Parliamentary and Health Service Ombudsman.

Ridgeway, V. (2011) 'Caring for the older person', M. Baldwin and J. Woodhouse (eds), *Key Concepts in Palliative Care*. London: Sage, pp. 26–30.

Royal College of Psychiatrists (2009) *No Health without Mental Health: The Supporting Evidence*. Available at: www.rcpsych.ac.uk/pdf/No%20Health%20-%20%20the%20 evidence_%20revised%20May%2010.pdf (accessed 4.6.15).

Saunders, C. (1976) 'Care of the dying', *Nursing Times*, 72(26): 1003–4.

Shuttleworth, A. (2005) 'Palliative care for people with end stage non-malignant lung disease', *Nursing Times*, 101(6): 48.

Skilbeck, J., Connor, J., Bath, P., Beech, N., Clark, D., Hughes, P., Douglas, H.R., Halliday, D., Haviland, J., Marples, R., Normand, C., Seymour, J. and Webb, T. (2002) 'A description of the Macmillan Nurse caseload. Part 1: Clinical nurse specialist in palliative care', *Palliative Medicine*, 16(4): 285–96.

Skilbeck, J.K. and Payne, S. (2005) 'End of life care: A discursive analysis of specialist palliative care nursing', *Journal of Advanced Nursing*, 51(4): 325–34.

Thomas, K. (2003) *Caring for the Dying at Home*. Abingdon: Radcliffe Medical Press.

Tilden, V.P. and Thompson, S. (1999) 'Policy issues in end-of-life care', *Journal of Professional Nursing*, 25(6): 363–8.

World Health Organization (1990) *Cancer Pain Relief and Palliative Care: Report of the WHO Expert Committee*. Geneva: WHO.

World Health Organization (2002) *National Cancer Control Programmes: Policies and Guidelines*. Geneva: WHO.

World Health Organization (2014) *Global Atlas of Palliative Care at the End of Life*. Geneva: WHO.

# 2

# Care and compassion in palliative care

---

This chapter will explore:

- compassion focused care and how it can facilitate the delivery of quality care
- how we can deliver that quality and ensure compassion is at the heart of the care we deliver
- the compassionate team approach
- how treating our colleagues and ourselves with compassion contributes to the quality of care we deliver to our patients and service users

---

## Quality care provision

Palliative care may be delivered by a range of health and social care professionals; for example, chaplains, occupational therapists, pharmacists and social workers. Support groups, including face-to-face and internet-based, are also available and may provide vital assistance and help to patients and their carers. Diversity within the team is essential as care needs may be complex and demanding. As professionals, we have a responsibility to ensure that the patient's journey and the carer's experience is cohesive and integrated using a compassionate, empathic approach where valuing the individual should be the philosophy underpinning all we do to care for a patient whilst incorporating effective communication with all those involved. If care is uncoordinated and patients and/or carers do not perceive consistent support, this may be significantly detrimental to their end of life care experience and may have a negative affect on our colleagues. As healthcare professionals we should be liaising with the team, and at the same time communicating with patients and their loved ones to ensure that the help and support they need is sufficient to ensure patient comfort and to help carers and relatives cope with the stressful and distressing journey that lies ahead of them. Patients' wishes at the end of life often include the intense need to ensure that their loved ones and carers receive support (whatever support may be needed) that incorporates empathy and compassion whilst caring for them and into bereavement (Richardson 2004).

## How can we provide quality in palliative care?

### 'No decision without me about me'

Ensuring the patient remains at the centre of all decision making and fostering the ideal of 'no decision without me about me' (DH 2012) is central to palliative care philosophy. Significant decisions may need to be made and could range from wishes surrounding preferred place of care (PPC) to more discreet choices concerning prioritising which symptom they would like dealing with first. Having informal carers involved in these decisions is also vital, as 'care partner' working becomes integral to the caring role (DH 2008).

Care, compassion, competence, communication, courage and commitment (known as 'the 6 Cs'; DH 2012) incorporate the excellence in care that we strive for as providers of that care (see Figure 2.1).

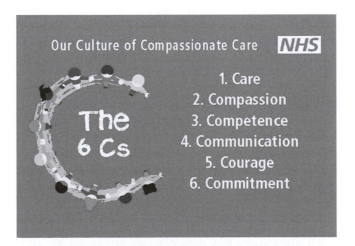

**Figure 2.1** The 6 Cs (Crown copyright)

At the end of 2012, the Department of Health issued the policy concerning compassion in practice. This policy is driven by staff, service users and key commissioning bodies wanting to see excellence in health and social care provision. They identified six key areas, as described below.

## Key area 1: Helping people to stay independent, maximising wellbeing and improving health outcomes

In palliative and end of life care, ensuring that symptom management is effective, and incorporating a holistic approach so that issues may be dealt with in a prompt and effective manner causing as little distress as possible, should be what we strive for as professionals (Ferrell and Coyle 2006). Maintaining as much independence as possible, no matter what the diagnosis, may aid and improve quality of life. One may argue that most people want to remain independent, being able to care for their own needs, being free to make decisions and maintain dignity. When a palliative or terminal phase diagnosis has been identified, trying to uphold independence for as long as possible is vital when time can be so limited.

---

 **Case scenario: John (part 1)**

John, 57, is a teacher and was admitted to hospital with acute bowel obstruction. He underwent surgical intervention and needed to have formation of a colostomy at the time of surgery. He was subsequently diagnosed with advanced colonic carcinoma. When he was 25 he had nursed his father who died of lung cancer aged 50. He felt his father died with very little dignity and suffered immensely. For John the priorities were to be able to care for his stoma independently and to continue to live life to the full, which included getting back to work. He needed to make decisions for himself, including those regarding any further treatment.

---

## Reflection points

- Which principles of key area 1 are embodied in this scenario?
- As a nurse, how can we help John?
- What about his father's death, do you think this might affect John's ability to deal with his illness?

---

Death anxiety as a phenomena has been extensively researched and debated. Even Plato, when drawing upon Socrates' argument, suggested that fearing death was wasted time as it is inevitable (Nicol and Nyatanga 2014). When a patient possesses disturbed or distressing experiences of death, this may have a negative impact on the way in which they deal with their own diagnosis and impending mortality. Talking about death and discussing John's fears about the way he dies may help to alleviate some of his concerns.

Death is generally misunderstood and a taboo subject within society. Dying Matters is a coalition set up by the National Council for Palliative Care to try to share thoughts and ideas about death, to reduce the mystique and misunderstanding and hopefully get people to talk, not only generally about death and dying but also to discuss and consider their own wishes at the end of life (Dying Matters 2015). They suggest that fearing death and not planning or considering one's own death is having a significant impact not only on the quality of life at the end of life but also the experience of death itself, with lack of support, lack of resources and failing to die in a place of one's choice. Death is inevitable and dismissing it and not speaking about it, as we know, does not defer the event itself. To ensure that people have access to compassionate care at the end of life, raising the subject and discussing their needs and wishes may facilitate high-quality care and a compassionate responsive approach may be used.

## Key area 2: Working with people to provide a positive experience of care.

Although repetitive, it is an overwhelming fact when caring for people with a life-limiting illness, time is limited by the nature of the diagnosis and to change a negative experience into a positive outcome may present a difficult challenge. What one can suggest is to eliminate these negative experiences completely. This may be idealistic, but to recognise one's own limitations and call for help is a responsibility we should be fostering as health and social care professionals. Working with people is crucial in palliative care as services involved may be diverse and communication between those services becomes essential for those receiving the service. It fosters trust and belief in those who are providing the care and support because care becomes focused and conflicting opinions and suggestions are limited as everyone strives for the same goals. The positive experience may be magnified if the patient receives excellent palliative and end of life care. They have care delivered by knowledgeable staff who are sensitive to both their needs and that of their carers. A companionship and collaborative approach is fostered and results in a more positive experience where a 'good death' may be achieved.

---

### 💬 Case scenario: John (part 2)

John declines any further treatment but would like symptomatic management of his condition. He currently experiences intermittent pain and this is limiting him somewhat. It is also a constant reminder of his diagnosis, which he chooses to ignore. John would like to stay at home and does not want any further admissions to hospital if possible.

*(Continued)*

*(Continued)*

His PPC is at home with his partner Derek. He was referred to the district nursing team and underwent a holistic assessment of his needs. Discussion regarding his current needs and wishes but also those at the end of life were discussed and documented. Both John and Derek had the opportunity to be involved in this discussion as Derek would be his primary carer. What was evident was that the pain had been difficult to control, and at the following visit the district nurse felt that both her and the general practitioner (GP) were struggling to regain the management of his pain, but also John now felt quite nauseous and anorexic. She contacted the Specialist Palliative Care team for their input. Following a couple of visits the team had made recommendations but also, more importantly, arranged contact should any further specialist input be required. The staff communicated regarding John's progress and determined that he was happy with his symptom management and felt that his quality of life had improved as a result of the interventions.

A partnership in caring was facilitated within all discussions and the visits thereafter. John had renewed faith in healthcare provision and felt much more empowered after discussing his experience with his father.

## Reflection points

- What principles of key area 2 are embodied in this scenario?
- How did the community team facilitate this?
- What skills and qualities do you feel are evident in this scenario?

## Key area 3: Delivering high-quality care and measuring the impact of care

High-quality care requires the input of staff who feel they want to give that level of care and who have the right knowledge and skills to not only deliver that care, but also differentiate between the standards that should and could be expected of the service providers. Understanding the support network available, resources, both equipment and expertise, understanding of the condition presenting as well as being able to carry out a comprehensive assessment of both the patient and the carer (DH 2008) should facilitate this high-quality care. Carers make a significant contribution to the delivery of care in the UK and abroad; valuing and supporting them, incorporating a compassionate philosophy of respect and empathy, kindness and trust has been identified as fundamental in the care of those with a life-limiting illness, especially those nursed in the community.

## Case scenario: John (part 3)

The district nursing team had a dedicated palliative care and end of life care champion who attended a number of study days but also ensured she networked with other staff, sharing expertise and case study discussions. She undertook post-registration education and completed a palliative care module at Masters level to facilitate and link her theory and practice skills. She became involved in John's care as it was recognised by the team that he would need a more knowledgeable practitioner. All the district nursing team had undertaken professional development in order to ensure that their practice was evidence based, in line with Nursing and Midwifery Council requirements (NMC 2015).

Discussions with John included informing him of support resources, offering referrals to a number of professionals that might assist both John and Derek (e.g. social workers for financial advice and help, occupational therapists to ensure that an appropriate and specialist assessment was undertaken). This allowed John and Derek to have access to equipment that might help John remain at home and facilitate not only John's but also Derek's safety, especially when considering moving and handling. The primary aim was to inform both John and Derek regarding the resources available and give them time to think about what they needed rather than to bombard them with information. The district nurse recognised that they were going through a traumatic time and would need all the team's support and help, both as a couple and as individuals with specific needs.

## Reflection points

- What key principles of key area 3 are embodied in this scenario?
- How did the community team facilitate this?
- What skills and qualities do you feel are evident in this scenario?
- How did they consider John's and Derek's needs?

## Key area 4: Building and strengthening leadership

So far the focus has been on teamwork; however, leadership also plays an important role in palliative care planning and provision. Understanding the significance of having a direction and goal in planning care at the end of life can be the difference between a cohesive team that achieves the patient's wishes and one that pulls in varying directions with little or nothing achieved, with the danger that the team may run out of time in trying to make a positive difference to that patient and their loved ones as they approach the end of life. Within the *Compassion in Practice* policy is the term 'emotional labour'(DH 2012). It considers the burden and distress that caring for vulnerable, sick and dying people can have on health and social care staff, and suggests that 'time and space is needed for individuals and teams to reflect, to share experiences and seek support and to build emotional resilience' (2012: 11).

---

### 👥 Case scenario: John (part 4)

The district nurse who conducted the initial assessment tried to maintain continuity with John and Derek as she and the team felt that this was important. So that everyone was familiar with the situation, however, after gaining consent from John and Derek she discussed the end of life plans with the immediate district nursing team and the GP. As other referrals were made (i.e. the social worker and the occupational therapist), they were given requisite information to help them in their assessment. This should always be on a need-to-know basis rather than disclosing everything (Caldicott 1997). As the number of visits and frequency increased, the district nurse also recognised the emotional strain this was having on both Derek and indeed on herself. She chose to ask for a meeting with her clinical supervisor to debrief and share some of her concerns (care was taken to maintain patient confidentiality throughout the session). After this she recognised that feeling emotionally drained was reasonable and she should not feel embarrassed or ashamed of this. She agreed with her supervisor to try to take part in an activity after work as this has been shown to benefit those with stress and anxiety (Melvin 2012) and to continue to attend for supervision sessions as it felt 'safe' when she shared her feelings.

---

### Reflection points

- What key principles of key area 4 are embodied in this scenario?
- How did the community team facilitate this?
- What do you think the district nurse's key qualities are?
- How do you think the clinical supervision sessions will help:

  o the district nurse?
  o John's and Derek's care?

- What important considerations did the district nurse make regarding John and Derek?

## Key area 5: Ensuring that we have the right staff, with the right skills, in the right place

Skilled staff are essential for effective palliative care delivery. Understanding the holistic needs of individuals at a time when they may undoubtedly be at their most vulnerable as a result of a life-changing as well as life-limiting diagnosis is fundamental. Once assessing and identifying key issues have been undertaken, the team then need to work with the patient and carer in trying to deal with symptoms, issues, anxiety and fears in a knowledgeable, understanding and effective manner, creating a belief and trust in the partnership.

 ## Case scenario: John (part 5)

The district nurse felt that the symptoms presented could be linked, but as time was limited and symptom management a priority she asked John if she could refer him to the specialist palliative care team (SPCT). Through this consultation and follow-up it was apparent that they were indeed linked and needed to be dealt with one by one rather than simply treating all the symptoms at once. This can negate and minimise the medication burden as with each drug given, possible interaction and reaction may occur. She contacted the SPCT and gained a great deal from their interventions, which she felt she could take forward and work on to improve her knowledge base. John and Derek were both extremely anxious about involving the SPCT and felt this meant that life was short, but she reassured them both that symptom management is part of the SPCT's role and expertise, and that this would not mean that they would continue to see the team but that they would be there if and when needed in the future. Although still a little anxious at the beginning of the consultation with the SPCT, when they completed the assessment and discussion, including asking what he thought about the treatments offered, John felt confident and reassured that he had been listened to and that together they would regain symptom control.

## Reflection points

- What key principles of key area 5 are embodied in this scenario?
- How did the community team facilitate this?
- What skills and qualities do you feel are evident in this scenario?
- How did the district nurse develop as a result of this interaction?

## Key area 6: Supporting positive staff experience

The significant and potentially detrimental effects of caring in an unsupported environment can mean the difference between quality care and that which falls far below a satisfactory level. Staff burnout, as Firth et al. (1986) suggested, may ensue from strain associated with emotive experiences and constant interaction with those who may be suffering themselves. This then results in significant psychological distress, with associated physical, spiritual and social symptoms.

> ### 📋 Case scenario: John (part 6)
>
> The district nursing team all support each other and take time to listen when they feel they are needed. They are a cohesive team and ensure that they know they can contact each other outside the working day if needed. During the morning, before visits, they ensure that they have time for each other and the wellbeing of each of them is everyone's business. The other district nurses recognised when John's main district nurse was becoming withdrawn. She appeared to be off her food and had little interest in meeting outside work. They carefully discussed how they were all feeling about John and Derek, giving the district nurse cues to share. As she started to share, they agreed that it was a difficult situation and that perhaps they could all seek some clinical supervision. This was an important point for the district nurse because she recognised that she was emotionally drained, and knowing that she was supported by her team was vital.

### Reflection points

- What key principles of key area 6 are embodied in this scenario?
- How did the community team facilitate this?
- What skills and qualities do you feel are evident in this scenario?
- How did they consider the district nurse's needs?
- How can this benefit the team?

## How can we improve our practice?

Examining the key targets allows one to establish the impact this policy could have on the patient, carer, relative and health and social care professional. What is needed now is to establish how these targets are to be met. One initiative that is being undertaken currently and may help to give us the 'how to' understanding has targeted cancer survivors specifically. The National Cancer Survivorship Initiative is a specialist team currently working to improve the quality of care by recruiting communities and piloting care strategies/models. This should provide frameworks that facilitate good practice and the consistency of practice for all who need cancer care and interventions. NICE also strive to create evidence-based guidance through robust research studies to inform practice (NICE 2011, 2012). What is needed is more research in the field of palliative and end of life care. In 2004, patient perceptions and end of life care were identified as a priority for more robust research and understanding. The National End of Life Care Intelligence Network (NEoLCIN) are addressing life-limiting illness and not just those with a cancer diagnosis; they are also examining the accessibility of palliative care to multiple social, economic and cultural groups (NEoLCIN 2011). The Network aims to examine quality, volume and cost of care provided by the NHS, social services and the third sector to adults approaching the end of life to help drive improvements in the quality and productivity of the care provided (Brown 2012).

The policies and guidance identified are a small number of those whose aim is to provide the framework for more coordinated, compassionate and responsive care which, for a person with a life-limiting illness, can be a relief and a great support. What is paramount and is reiterated in the palliative and end of life care strategies is the requirement that the care people receive as they are dealing with a life-limiting illness is aligned to their needs and preferences and delivered with compassion. What we need to be clear about is what is compassion and how do we display it?

Compassion involves wanting to understand and trying to identify people's feelings, emotions and needs. Self-compassion involves understanding and identifying our own emotions, feelings and needs. Ignoring or failing to recognise either our own need or that of someone in our care means we are negatively affecting our capacity for compassion. A distancing exercise occurs between ourselves and those we are supposed to be helping and caring for, which can lead to feelings of mistrust in the patient and carer (Doyle and Jeffrey 2000). To be compassionate involves engaging in empathy, wanting to care, to do the best one can, wanting to understand the issues and be interested and positively affect a patient's wellbeing. Without this engagement and desire to understand, compassion may be lost and with that, trust, quality and detailed attention. This will have a negative effect on any person in need of care. A patient who may be approaching the end of life deserves better than sub-optimal care.

The key attribute in aiding compassionate care is competent communication skills. Without the ability to communicate effectively, engagement with the patient and their carer becomes fraught with issues, including misunderstanding and misinterpretation. Carers were interviewed in Lee's study (2002). Poor communication predisposed the carer and patient to dreadful experiences, therefore with enhanced communication skills a therapeutic relationship may be developed that is embedded in compassionate care. Compassion and effective communication should be synonymous with all those we have contact with, including those we work alongside, to ensure a harmonious, supportive environment where one does not feel judged.

## The team approach

Palliative care is delivered in numerous environments by a variety of staff with varying experience. In some circumstances, the disease or situation itself may be extremely complex and the specialist palliative care team may be called upon for their expertise in palliative and end of life care. The team often consists of a range of professionals who work together for the benefit of the patient and their carer. This teamwork comes with a range of expertise as well as a mutual recognition regarding each others' contribution to care provision. Rationale for referral to a specialist palliative care team may be comprehensive and multidimensional, therefore having a cohesive team to help support the professionals already involved and patients and carers may be invaluable.

Unfortunately, referrals to specialist teams may be as a result of perceived inadequacy. This can culminate in a lack of understanding or lack of knowledge and may be combined with a lack of preparedness or inability to deal with the emotional burden. Failing to respond to these negative feelings will only exacerbate the perceptions and result in patient suffering (Davies 2003). What is evident is that a uniform approach to palliative and end of life care should be adopted, and that listening, informing and referring to other members of the multidisciplinary team when appropriate can all aid the best possible quality of life and facilitate a compassionate approach to end of life care (Brown 2012). Davies (2003) reported a mixed response in the literature to professional caring, especially when the patients have extremely distressing symptoms. She cited Menzies' research (1970), who suggested that the caring role created a huge number of feelings and experiences and that when examining these, it is apparent that some situations present conflict for the professional carer (e.g. resentment versus compassion). Davitz and Davitz (1975) reported more helplessness and feelings of inadequacy, whilst Field (1984) focused specifically on end of life care and the participants in his study suggested the rewards were clear when delivering end of life care, culminating in an opportunity to implement gold-standard nursing care. This research highlights the challenges palliative and end of life care present. It may also provide an opportunity to use one's skills and knowledge and have a positive impact when caring for those with a life-limiting illness.

## The cost of caring

Palliative and end of life care may be a distressing experience. Psychological and social distress may ensue as a result of a life that is limited. Dreams, plans and the future become more uncertain as a diagnosis of a life-limiting condition is delivered. This may leave the patient and their loved ones in a distressed state, not knowing what to do or how to share their feelings. Fear regarding the journey ahead and the outcome that journey may have all add to the devastation that the diagnosis has for everyone involved. Treatments may be enduring and, whilst distressing for the patient, leave informal carers and loved ones with a slightly different distress. This may encompass feelings of helplessness, lack of understanding, uncertainty and nauseating anxiety (Sheldon 2003). In addition to this extensive suffering, relatives and friends may be struggling with the thought of losing their loved one even before the loss. Healthcare professionals therefore need to support and be compassionate, not only with the patient but with the family and loved ones. Without this support, they may feel that they are unable to cope with what the future holds, and this may have a negative impact on any future end of life experience (see Chapter 5 for further discussion surrounding the burden of care).

# Compassion and self-compassion

Ferrell and Coyle (2006) identified that patients at the end of life should receive 'exquisite care', but this level of care may have significant demands on those providing it as it requires compassion and empathy at its core and these can be attributes which, if not replenished, can lead to potentially harmful consequences. Nurses in the position of caring for all involved may themselves find this daunting and emotionally and physically exhausting, which should be recognised. Self-compassion and recognising one's own stress and anxiety helps us to identify stress and anxiety in others (see Chapter 11 for further discussion). Several negative effects have been identified when undertaking prolonged caring, especially for those with a distressing illness, which include professional compassion fatigue, burnout and accumulated loss phenomena (Melvin 2012). Cole-King and Gilbert (2011) tried to establish what constitutes compassion and suggested it consisted of empathy, warmth, being kind to others, and a non-judgmental approach. Davison and Williams (2009) called for more clarity regarding compassion, including what it looks like, how to measure it and for more debate, in the hope that it can be fostered and embedded in all nursing care.

There are undoubtedly considerable benefits in caring for a patient; the privilege it holds is immeasurable, but the greater the time in formal caring for those in this distressed state, the more chance that the individual may become affected psychologically, spiritually, physically, emotionally and/or socially (Showalter 2010). Health and social care professionals need to be aware of the resources available for the patients, informal carers and themselves, and in addition have an awareness of current evidence, including any policies or frameworks which inform or regulate practice. Failure to manage oneself and care for others adequately may result in unjustifiable suffering, culminating in significant consequences for those involved (Davies 2003).

In today's health and social care provision when atrocities like Mid Stafford and Winterbourne are being reported, one must ask how compassion is being facilitated. Are nurses dealing with their conflicts? Is 'helplessness' and 'inadequacy' in conflict with the delivery of compassionate care? Compassion has been recognised as a significant and essential requirement when caring for a patient, but also to be compassionate one perhaps needs to be compassionate with oneself. The final chapter of this book will focus on self-compassion and how one may recognise emotional conflict and burden, as conflict, burden and burnout can have a negative effect on the care delivered.

Reflecting on situations and recognising when one needs to seek support and help is vital, not only for the wellbeing of those in our care but also for the wellbeing of ourselves and our colleagues. This recognition is a strength, not a weakness, and will allow us to continue to provide the compassionate care we strive to deliver every day.

# Conclusion

This chapter has highlighted the need for education and support to staff providing palliative and end of life care. Further staff development and support are needed to help integrate the six key areas identified by the DH (2012) into practice and see a significant improvement in the quality of care for all no matter what the diagnosis, gender, age, culture, geographical area or socioeconomic background. The aim is to ensure that patients are empowered and feel that staff providing their care are responsive to their needs, and that investment is needed in all staff no matter what profession or place of care provision. In addition, caring for each other and displaying compassionate attitudes to those we work alongside should be harnessed in order to provide a supportive, healthy environment. With an increasingly aging population who are reported to be the largest consumers of healthcare resources (DH 2001), greater demands on services may be encountered, and the effective means of managing symptoms and caring with compassion and commitment will be essential for those in the palliative and terminal phase of illness. Prioritising patients' wishes and needs creates a responsive approach, which is what we should all strive for.

## Reflection points

Think about the last patient you cared for:

- How did you facilitate a compassionate approach?
- How did this help the patient?
- How did this help the relatives?
- How do you facilitate compassion for your colleagues?
- How can you be compassionate to yourself?

## Suggested reading

Cole-King, A. and Gilbert, P. (2011) 'Compassionate care: The theory and the reality', *Journal of Holistic Healthcare*, 8(3): 29–36.
Davies, H. (2003) 'The emotional load of caring: Care for those for whom there is no cure', in B. Nyatanga and M. Astley-Pepper (eds), *Hidden Aspects of Palliative Care*. London: Quay Books.
Department of Health (2012) *Compassion in Practice*. London: HMSO.

## References

Brown, M. (2012) 'Care and compassion at the end of life', *Journal of Care Services Management*, 6(2): 69–73.
Caldicott, F. (1997) *Report on the Review of Patient-identifiable Information: The Caldicott Committee*. London: DH.
Cole-King, A. and Gilbert, P. (2011) 'Compassionate care: The theory and the reality', *Journal of Holistic Healthcare*, 8(3): 29–36.

Davies, H. (2003) 'The emotional load of caring: Care for those for whom there is no cure', in B. Nyatanga and M. Astley-Pepper (eds), *Hidden Aspects of Palliative Care*. London: Quay Books.

Davison, N. and Williams, K. (2009) 'Compassion in nursing 1: Defining, identifying and measuring this essential quality', *Nursing Times*, 14 September.

Davitz, J.R. and Davitz, L.J. (1975) 'How do nurses feel when patients suffer?', *American Journal of Nursing*, 75(9): 1505–10.

Department of Health (2001) *National Service Framework for Older People: Executive Summary*. London: HMSO.

Department of Health (2008) *End of Life Care Strategy*. London: HMSO.

Department of Health (2012) *Compassion in Practice*. London: HMSO.

Doyle, D. and Jeffrey, D. (2000) *Palliative Care in the Home*. York: Oxford University Press.

Dying Matters (2015) *Raising Awareness of Dying, Death and Bereavement*. Available at: http://dyingmatters.org/overview/about-us (accessed 4.6.15).

Ferrell, B. and Coyle, N. (2006) *Oxford Textbook of Palliative Nursing*, 2nd edn. New York: Oxford University Press.

Field, D. (1984) "We didn't want him to die on his own": Nurses' accounts of nursing dying patients', *Journal of Advanced Nursing*, 9: 59–70.

Firth, H., McIntee, J., McKeown, P. and Britton, P. (1986) 'Burnout and professional depression: Related concepts?', *Journal of Advanced Nursing*, 11: 633–41.

Lee, E. (2002) *In Your Own Time: A Guide for Patients and their Carers Facing a Last Illness at Home*. Oxford: Oxford University Press.

Melvin, C. (2012) 'Professional compassion fatigue: What is the true cost of nurses caring for the dying?', *International Journal of Palliative Nursing*, 18(12): 606–11.

Menzies, E.P. (1970) *The Functioning of Social Systems as a Defence Against Anxiety*. London: Tavistock.

National End of Life Care Intelligence Network (2011) Predicting Death: Estimating the Proportion of Deaths that are 'Unexpected'. Bristol: National End of Life Care Intelligence Network. Available at: www.endoflifecare-intelligence.org.uk/view?rid=116 (accessed 4.6.15).

National Institute for Health and Care Excellence (2011) *Quality Standard for End of Life Care for Adults*. London: NICE.

National Institute for Health and Care Excellence (2012) *Opioids in Palliative Care: Safe and Effective Prescribing of Strong Opioids for Pain in Palliative Care of Adults*. London: NICE.

Nicol, J. and Nyatanga, B. (2014) *Palliative and End of Life Care in Nursing*. London: Sage.

Nursing and Midwifery Council (2015) *The Code: Professional Standards of Practice and Behaviour for Nurses and Midwives*. London: NMC.

Richardson, A. (2004) 'Creating a culture of compassion: Developing supportive care for people with cancer', *European Journal of Oncology*, 8: 293–305.

Sheldon, F. (2003) 'Social impact of advanced cancer', in M. Lloyd-Williams (ed.), *Psychosocial Issues in Palliative Care*. Oxford: Oxford University Press.

Showalter, S. (2010) 'Compassion fatigue: What is it? Why does it matter? Recognising the symptoms, acknowledging the impact, developing the tools to prevent compassion fatigue, and strengthen the professional already suffering the effects', *American Journal of Hospice and Palliative Medicine*, 27(4): 239–42.

# 3

# Holistic assessment

## Michelle Brown and Kersten Hardy

This chapter will explore:

- holistic assessment and holistic care
- the interprofessional team and its contribution to holistic care
- the key requirements for effective holistic care and assessment
- assessment tools and the benefits of utilising the tools available
- research in palliative care, indicating the difficulties inherent in recruiting and conducting a study with this vulnerable group of patients.

## What is a holistic approach?

As a healthcare professional it is a pertinent skill to be able to assess, plan, implement and evaluate the fundamental needs of patients in your care. This is to ensure that the care they receive is effective, but primarily based upon maintaining dignity, compassion and promoting a more positive personal experience of being a patient.

The assessment of a patient with palliative care needs requires a comprehensive, structured approach (Payne et al. 2008), with full consideration to not only the presenting need but also all aspects of daily living; this is referred to as the 'holistic approach'. Holistic care is often viewed as the active care of patients and requires the assessor to not only consider the patient's functional ability, but also to individualise care by exploring, in depth, the patients physical, social, psychological, emotional and spiritual needs (see Figure 3.1).

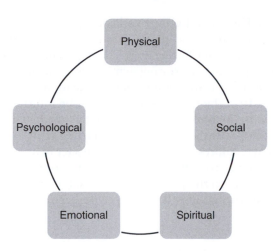

**Figure 3.1** Holistic care

The Department of Health (2008, 2009) have, inadvertently, determined that the care delivered should exceed the holistic domains identified by Payne et al. (2008) but should also incorporate the cultural, environmental and financial elements of daily living. Although essentially these arenas form the basis of a holistic assessment and the delivery of holistic care, it is important to understand how these may affect the patient and, as an assessor, how to apply them to individualised care delivery. The National Cancer Action Team (NCAT 2012) identified the benefits of holistic assessment and suggest that it has a significant impact on the patient's experience and can help to improve outcomes as it allows a more proactive and responsive approach to patient care. Henoch et al. (2011) examined quality of life in patients with a cancer diagnosis. They identified that poor mental health functioning can have a significant effect on overall quality of life, therefore to simply address physical domains will fail to address the issues which may be contributing to their distress (see Figure 3.2).

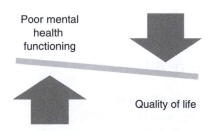

**Figure 3.2** Quality of life in cancer patients (Henoch et al. 2011)

National Institute for Health and Care Excellence guidance (2011) emphasises the importance of managing both the physical and psychological needs of patients approaching the end of life and further suggests employing any available resources to help address and treat any distressing symptoms or problems and to optimise their comfort (e.g. specialist teams, equipment, medication).

Issues which may affect the patient's journey can be multifaceted and be either intrinsic or extrinsic or a combination, but what is evident is that they will, at some point, affect the patient's experience or journey with some degree of positive or negative impact. Addressing the negative impact in any of these domains at assessment is crucial in improving the patient's quality of life; what may appear to some as unimportant can, to the patient, be the basis of anxiety and fear, possibly exacerbating other issues that may have otherwise been easily dealt with.

## The patient at the centre

The holistic assessment should be patient-centred with adequate time given for the patient to gain trust in the assessor, thus giving the opportunity for the patient to fully express their needs and concerns (NCAT 2012, 2015). With this empowerment and relationship, the patient may be able to make some decisions for future care and, if appropriate at the time, the preferred options for their end of life care (see Chapters 8 and 9 for further discussion) (NHS 2004; NEoLCP 2015; NICE 2004).

Consideration should always be made to current evidence-based practice when supporting the patient through the holistic assessment, and the assessor should seek to address the patient's and carer's concerns in a collaborative manner. As the patient and carer begin to prioritise elements of care and problems that are important to them, it is essential to plan with them how these issues can honestly be addressed. It is important to be aware that the priorities, choices and decisions made by the individual will be a constantly changing agenda as experiences and situations may have an impact on the patient's journey (i.e. an acute change in condition) (DH 2008, 2009). As the patient approaches the end of life phase, the patient's wishes surrounding place of care/death could change, from being at home to being in hospital or a hospice environment. Two pertinent examples of this change in plan are fear and support.

 **Case scenario: Adam**

Adam is 60 and has end stage COPD, he has discussed his care with the specialist nurse and his family and planned to have his end of life care at home. Adam then suffered an exacerbation of his illness and developed pneumonia. He was admitted to hospital for treatment, but it soon became evident that Adam had entered the terminal phase of his COPD. He is now struggling to breathe and needs oxygen continually.

He is frightened about his difficulty in breathing and despite the good symptom management he has decided that he does not want to be at home. He feels safe and secure in the hospital environment, but does not want to upset his family as he feels that being at home would not be the right place for him.

## Reflection points

- How can we be sure that Adam truly feels this is right for him?
- Think about Adam and how he may feel: can you see why he may have changed his mind?
- Is there anything you think we could do to support him further?
- How can we support Adam regarding his breathlessness and significant fear of taking his last breath?

What we want today may not be what we want tomorrow, therefore holistic care should involve regular reassessment, planning, implementation and evaluation in order to ensure that the care delivered is current and relevant to the patient's changing needs (NCAT 2012). Breathlessness is an extremely distressing state, and as nurses we need to ensure that the patient is supported and that all available treatment to reduce breathlessness is undertaken; for example, psychological support may be given by reassuring and openly acknowledging the fear of breathlessness, as well as relaxation therapies that attempt to control breathing, fan therapy, positioning, bronchodilator drugs (nebuliser or inhaler delivered) and opiates in very low doses as they reach the end of life (2.5–5 mg as needed) (Twycross and Wilcock 2001).

## Holistic assessment and patient understanding

As identified by a number of significant publications that the World Health Organization (2007, 2014) has developed, holistic care is not restricted to end of life care in the UK; it is an international priority. Pederson and Emmers-Sommer (2012) suggested that there is very little understanding of holistic care from a patient's point of view. In their study they interviewed ten patients who had advanced disease and were being cared for under either a hospice or home programme, and all of the participants identified the care interventions they had received using a biomedical approach. It was evident that they had little understanding of how their care needs were being met using a holistic philosophy. This could have a negative effect on the patient, with a failure to address anxieties or issues that they deem unimportant or not part of the healthcare professional's remit. The outcome of this study identified that there is a significant question regarding the approach that healthcare professionals have to consider when caring for the individual. Is it clear that we are caring for them as a 'whole person?' Do they understand what we mean by a 'whole person', and do we need to make that distinction? It is quite possible that if the healthcare professional was to stress that the aim was to not only meet their physical needs but also to address all of the domains associated with holism, then this might promote a feeling of safety and reassurance that they are being heard. It may also provide the patient with a perceived permission to discuss any issues that are concerning them rather than only those that they feel are of relevance which, judging by the latter research study, may be predominantly physical concerns.

## Symptoms and the holistic approach

It is important to understand that holistic care means that we recognise a problem but do not isolate it to simply a physical problem or psychological issue. An example of this would be fatigue in a patient with a gastric carcinoma. Lack of nutrition and appetite would contribute to fatigue and could be identified as physical issues, but fatigue could also be contributed to by the patient's emotional and psychological state. The patient may be worrying about the future, about the physical symptoms or they may be feeling low in mood, which has been identified as a relatively common experience for those with a life-limiting illness. It is therefore quite clear that a multidimensional approach is imperative in helping and responding to the complex needs a patient may have (DH 2010).

A study completed by Johnsen et al. (2009) explored the impact of specialist palliative care and the holistic assessment of symptoms related to patients with advanced cancer. They noted that one domain overlapped another. They also identified that divorced or widowed patients had more appetite loss than those who were married or single. The physical symptom of a poor appetite therefore can be affected by the social and psychological factors.

The holistic assessment is closely linked with the delivery of holistic care, as the ability to deliver and promote interventions is just as important as the assessment. Holistic care encompasses all attributes of daily living, from bathing, dressing, eating, talking, listening, being able to comfort, reassure and provide relief for all clinical needs from managing elimination to the delivery of regular and rescue medications. This does not mean the overall ability to administer the multitude of medications required for the management of symptoms, but rather to have the confidence and competence to deliver the myriad treatments and interventions which are prescribed and planned for, with the aim of meeting the patient's potential plethora of needs. It is important to be aware that the delivery of palliative care and holism is constantly developing; the stress of being up to date with current practice and being aware of the absolute latest evidence-based knowledge in palliative care has never been so pertinent to healthcare professionals (HCPs) and patients (DH 2010). It is fair to say that currently we are living in an increasingly aging population; we are living longer, even with life-limiting conditions such as COPD, heart failure, motor neurone disease and cancer (Kaspers et al. 2012). It is because of this and the advances in research that we are now nursing palliative care patients with increasingly complex needs (Kaspers et al. 2012). The profusion of treatments available to maintain dignity and control symptoms has developed to ensure that patients who move into the palliative stage of illness should not fear inadequately controlled symptoms, a diminished quality of life and/or a 'bad death' (Duffy 2011). Such interventions could include the expertise from other members of the interprofessional team (see Figure 3.3).

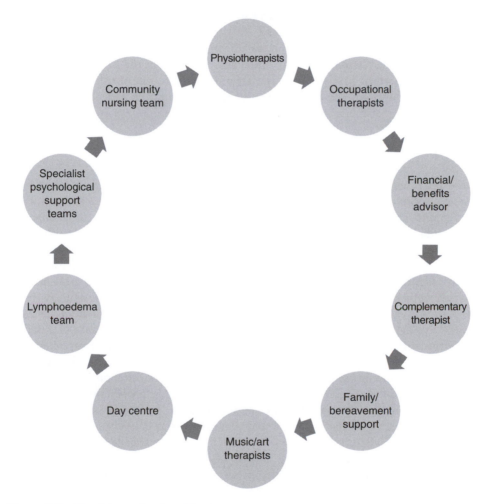

**Figure 3.3**  The interprofessional team

These may include physiotherapists, occupational therapists, financial/benefit advisor, complimentary therapists, musical/art therapists, family/bereavement support teams, psychological support teams, day-centres, lymphoedema teams and community nursing teams for example. The resources are extensive and can make a significant difference to patient and carer wellbeing. Referrals to physiotherapists and occupational therapists can promote the patient's independence as mobility aids and adaptive methods can be introduced to empower the patient in maintaining control, which in turn can have significant impact on their psychological wellbeing. This may aid the carer and keep them from harm, but also give them reassurance at a time where they may be feeling overwhelmed by the level of personal care they are delivering to their loved one. So consideration is not only made to the patient's physical need within the holistic assessment, but it should also involve the patient's psychosocial requirements and that of their carer's. The holistic assessment and interventions implemented require effective listening skills to ensure that the issues have been interpreted correctly. The utilisation of effective listening skills when providing holistic care can also enhance therapeutic engagement with the patient (Payne et al. 2008). It is important to also consider that a therapeutic relationship will promote trust and the ability for the patient to share their confidences with the HCP.

## The links between the health domains

As the HCP begins to understand how one symptom overlaps another, affecting at least one more arena of daily living, it becomes quite clear that they all have a significant impact on the patient's psychological and social status. It is often reported from studies within palliative care that psychological care is the least addressed within the health and social care environment, yet it is linked in one way or another to all the arenas of daily living (Johnston and Smith 2006). Unfortunately some studies have identified that little can be done to alter the patient's psychological need, as results have demonstrated that low mood and depression go hand in hand with not only terminal cancer, but also just the diagnosis of cancer whether potentially curable or palliative (Massie 2004). This finding is of concern as the aim for care of a patient is to optimise quality of life and eventually facilitate a good death. It is important that the patient's psychological wellbeing is given the attention it deserves and is reviewed in a holistic manner in an endeavour to ensure an optimum outcome for the patient. The abundance of local and national policies reiterate that patients with cancer and other life-limiting conditions should be supported in all levels of psychological need, but in order to achieve this it is suggested that an enhanced level of communication is key to effectively support patients. It is fair to say that excellent communication skills are essential in completing the holistic assessment for a palliative care patient as a whole, due to the sensitive but also proactive approach needed.

## Knowledge as a need

It is clear that, in order to complete a holistic assessment, we need not only the knowledge of the complex symptoms that can present in a patient with a life-limiting condition, but also knowledge of how these symptoms can overlap and affect all arenas of daily living. It is imperative that the holistic assessment and holistic care is delivered by the interprofessional team to ensure that the patient is offered a choice of comprehensive approaches and options (NCAT 2012). Once again, here is where excellent communication skills are required to ensure effective communication between teams, as this is fundamental in making sure that a seamless approach is fostered (see Chapter 6).

## Spiritual care

When considering the interprofessional team it is important to offer a spiritualist or chaplain, as historically a patient's spiritual needs have received little recognition within healthcare provision unless a patient is actively practicing in their chosen faith. The spiritual needs of a patient have been actively researched by some, possibly in an attempt to understand how to support the individual's spiritual needs, but can frequently be left by the professional as an issue for other team members to deal with, primarily the chaplain (DH 2010). We must recognise, however, that spirituality is more than religious faith: it is who we are as a person, what we feel we represent, and therefore this may be at risk when a patient is presented with an advancing life-limiting illness because their role and responsibilities may be constrained by the disease and its complications or enduring symptoms. It is a pertinent aspect of the patient's journey and should be fully included within the holistic assessment, as this is a significant element to future care wishes and an important part of the role of any HCP involved with a patient who has a life-limiting condition.

## Honesty and decision making

Ultimately to provide holistic care, it is imperative that the clinician is able to consider life-limiting illness trajectories and use this knowledge to apply the holistic assessment to each individual (Sallnow et al. 2012). Lack of understanding could have a significant impact on the patient's journey, as this may allow the reality of their prognosis to remain imprudent, encouraging the patient and their loved ones to fight for life until death. Caution must be taken when discussing future care, however, as the risk of erasing any hope they may have could cause psychological decline, which may result in a poor quality of life. But in turn, for the patient to live with quality and to be fully empowered in any decisions regarding their life, it is morally important to be open and honest as this is acquiescent to a true prognosis. This could prevent the patient from asking for inappropriate aggressive interventions that will have little impact on their prognosis but would be likely to contribute to a negative impact on their quality of life if undertaken (Ahlner-Elmqvist et al. 2009). Although a patient cannot demand treatments, when a patient has unrealistic expectations it could lead to a difficult consultation and may cause distress to all concerned, particularly the patient and their loved ones. Open dialogue can also help the patient to plan ahead and make choices should they need to. A family disagreement resulting in estranged relationships, an important event, a secret that needs to be shared may all be addressed if one is aware of the prognosis.

## The effective discussion

It is clear that there are a number of principles that help underpin holism; if these are carefully considered, it will enable the HCP to undertake a purposeful holistic assessment. To begin with the HCP will require an in-depth understanding surrounding the domains that may have an impact on the patient's wellbeing: these are physical, psychological, spiritual, social, cultural, environmental and financial. There may be intrinsic and extrinsic factors which have a further impact on the patient. These could include the provision of services, available resources, previous experiences, existing relationships and support mechanisms available. This knowledge integrated with the activities of daily living (e.g. eating and drinking, elimination, washing and dressing) should enable the HCP to consider and prompt the patient to discuss problems or issues that could develop and may not otherwise have been considered in addition to the actual presenting problem (NCAT 2012). Also, the HCP must be able to demonstrate excellent communication and interprofessional skills in order to address problems expressed by the patient. Understanding how an arena could interlink with one or more others is essential in meeting the patient's needs, either by referral to other teams or by the simple task of care planning. The awareness of disease trajectories is significant when planning the care with a patient; a knowledgeable yet open and honest approach will help empower the patient, thus facilitating trust and a feeling of safety. Together these principles alongside the simple nursing review of 'assess, plan, implement and evaluate' will enable the holistic assessment to take place, which in turn should facilitate the delivery of holistic care. It is important to remember that a patient who has palliative care needs at the end of life will have an ever changing agenda, and will depend highly on mood, anxieties and current capabilities. This will require the HCP to support and advise the patient further, initiating the assessment, planning, implementing and evaluating care as needed.

Applying this knowledge to a patient who is in the palliative phase of their illness will facilitate a comprehensive holistic assessment and promote the delivery of holistic care. This skill is transferable and is recommended for all patients receiving medical care (Sallnow et al. 2012), and with practice will become the basis of any assessment a HCP may make with a patient. Consider how you would assess the patient in the following case study.

 **Case scenario: Jane**

Jane is 45 and has ovarian cancer, with liver metastases; she has a very supportive family who wish to be actively involved with her care delivery. She presents with a cachexic (emaciated and malnourished) appearance to her upper body, but has bilateral leg oedema which is slowly spreading up into her lower body. Her verbalised complaints are nausea and vomiting and feeling short of breath when walking.

## Reflection points

- What potential problems can you anticipate from Jane's presenting condition?
- What support or referral can you offer Jane and her family?
- How can you facilitate holistic care?
- Think of a situation where holistic care helped a patient who you felt was suffering.
- Think how you can develop your skills to improve your care delivery.

Although this may all be idealistic, we should still strive for excellence. Issues and factors may hinder the holistic assessment process, for example lack of knowledge and understanding of the healthcare or social care professional, and failure to identify when a person is reaching the end of life, which limits the time for discussion surrounding anxieties, wishes and needs. The challenges to delivering holistic care are numerous. Recognising our own limitations is crucial to the process, therefore seeking help from other professionals or accessing further education should be paramount. Lack of recognition surrounding the dying phase can mean that the assessment of those at the end of life fails to address all aspects or issues due to lack of time, not only for the assessment but also to carry out any required interventions and treatments. This may present a dilemma as we need to complete a full and comprehensive assessment, but if a patient is too ill or fatigued we may need to prioritise issues to be addressed first and foremost, with a further, more robust exploration and discussion at a later date. One may argue that to start a full assessment and not complete it due to a patient's deteriorating health is better than to not start it at all.

## A guide to the assessment and tools available

To promote holistic care and the holistic assessment a number of assessment tools can be utilised. Unfortunately, these are predominantly generic and are not always appropriate in palliative care. Three common tools adopted to help either to assess a patient or to know when they need more specialist support are the Distress Thermometer (National Comprehensive Cancer Network 2013), PEPSI COLA aide memoire (Thomas 2003) and the Sheffield Profile for Assessment and Referral for Care (SPARC) (Ahmedzai and Noble 2007).

The Distress Thermometer is a tool that uses a picture of a thermometer alongside a tick-box list, which requires the patient to consider any symptoms or problems they have and place them in order of priority against the thermometer, which should help to identify specific needs but also if a patient presents with significant deterioration and needs a more rapid approach to their assessment, then this may facilitate that, ensuring that the patient's priorities are not lost in the assessment process. The PEPSI COLA aide memoire is based on prompting the assessor to consider aspects of daily living. The SPARC tool was introduced to help healthcare professionals identify when patients need specialist palliative care referral. It was acknowledged that equity of palliative care resources was in question and identified as a public health issue (Ahmedzai and Noble 2007).

## The Distress Thermometer

The Distress Thermometer requires the patient's input, but could easily be adapted for use when assessing a patient at an in-patient unit. The Distress Thermometer has several variations which verify its ability to be used in differing environments of care delivery. It differs from the other tools in that it is not designed for patient self-assessment, so could prove beneficial for the HCP to use within a hospital environment.

## PEPSI COLA aide memoire

The acronym PEPSI COLA is construed from physical, emotional, personal, social support, information/communication, control, out of hours, living with your illness and after care. These word prompts enable the assessor to consider the whole person, elicit other areas of potential problems and apply them with the patient to the plan of care (See Chapter 9 for further discussion).

## SPARC

SPARC is a tool which encompasses an introductory and explanatory paragraph, followed by 45 questions. The questions work through seven aspects of patient need, which require the patient to score how they have been affected by symptoms related to life-limiting conditions during the last month.

## The benefits and disadvantages of tools

Although these tools are useful in helping with the holistic assessment and in relation to all types of assessment tools, they have positive and negative implications. SPARC, for example, was developed in Sheffield and designed for use with patients with all types of life-limiting conditions, which is of benefit when considering equity of access, but it was introduced as a trigger for referral to specialist teams rather than for carrying out a holistic assessment and forming treatment plans and strategies.

It is clear with each tool that to enable the patient to gain any positive impact, the assessor should be able to clearly explain its use and effectiveness, along with the patient having not only the capacity to use it but also the energy levels to complete the tool (NCAT 2012, 2015). This is essentially where the assessor should have the skill and knowledge to complete a holistic assessment without the need for prompts and tools. Although the three tools described briefly above are designed to help with the holistic assessment of a patient with a life-limiting illness, they are not specifically designed for use within the palliative stage of illness.

## Research and palliative care

Assessment tools are often discussed and debated for use within palliative care – pain scores and delirium assessments are pertinent examples. It is often identified that specific tools for palliative care patients are not appropriate due to the ethics that surround establishing substantiated results. Research is difficult in palliative care as attrition (patients failing to complete the study due to deterioration) or recruiting significant sample sizes may be difficult, alongside the fear of whether it is ethically and morally right to burden a patient as they reach the end of life with questions and tools. Therefore we are left asking whether we have valid, robust tools that meet patients' needs. Where necessary research is granted, as it can be argued at times that the participation in research can propel treatments and new practices for the greater good forward (Stevens et al. 2003; Dean and McClement 2002). Where this is the situation, questionnaires and assessment tools are, where possible, kept simplistic and user friendly (Dean and McClement 2002). Preconceptions regarding the appropriateness of research in patients who are either palliative or at the end of their life have been argued by Alexander (2010), who states that there is no clear evidence to suggest patient harm or increased distress but argues that the constructive impact of participation outweighs any negativity as the progression of treatment is advancing as a result. What one should be assured of is that the patient has the capacity to understand the undertaking and is fully informed of their role and the requirements the study has.

## Conclusion

This chapter has explored the approach in effectively completing the holistic assessment of a patient within your care who is in the palliative stage of their illness. It is intended to provide a basis of how to apply holism to your daily nursing care delivery, but with the intention that it will encourage you to explore it in depth to continue your development and knowledge base. The exploration of holistic assessment tools, although brief, has clarified that even with the use of such tools; the assessor still requires excellent communication skills and knowledge of all arenas of daily living in order to ensure a full holistic assessment, which will in turn reward you with the ability to meet the patient's needs fully.

## Suggested reading

Duffy, S. (2011) *Dying with Dignity: Applying Personalisation to End of Life Care*. London: Centre for Welfare Reform. Available at: www.centreforwelfarereform.org/uploads/attachment/296/dying-with-dignity.pdf (accessed 4.6.15).

National Cancer Action Team (2012) *Holistic Needs Assessment for People with Cancer: A Practical Guide for Healthcare Professionals*. London: NCAT. Available at: www.ncsi. org.uk/wp-content/uploads/The_holistic_needs_assessment_for_people_with_cancer_A_ practical_Guide_NCAT.pdf (accessed 4.6.15).

National Institute for Health and Care Excellence (2011) *Quality Standard for End of Life Care in Adults*. London: NICE. Available at: www.nice.org.uk/guidance/qs13/chapter/ quality-statement-5-holistic-support-social-practical-and-emotional (accessed 4.6.15).

# References

Ahlner-Elmqvist, M., Bjordal, K., Jordhey, M.S., Kaasa, S. and Jannert, M. (2009) 'Characteristics and implications of attrition in health-related quality of life studies in palliative care', *Palliative Medicine*, 23(5): 432–40.

Ahmedzai, S. and Noble, B. (2007) *Sheffield Profile for Assessment and Referral for Care*. Available at: www.ncsi.org.uk/wp-content/uploads/SPARC-Assessment-Tool.pdf (accessed 4.6.15).

Alexander, S.J. (2010) 'As long as it helps somebody: Why vulnerable people participate in research', *International Journal of Palliative Nursing*, 16(4): 174–9.

Dean, R.A. and McClement, S.E. (2002) 'Palliative care research: Methodological and ethical challenges', *International Journal of Palliative Nursing*, 8(8): 246–380.

Department of Health (2008) *End of Life Care Strategy: Promoting High Quality Care for all Adults at the End of Life*. London: HMSO.

Department of Health (2009) *End of Life Care Strategy: Quality Markers and Measures for End of Life Care*. London: HMSO.

Department of Health (2010) *Improving Outcomes: A Strategy for Cancer*. London: HMSO.

Duffy, S. (2011) *Dying with Dignity: Applying Personalisation to End of Life Care*. London: Centre for Welfare Reform. Available at: www.centreforwelfarereform.org/uploads/ attachment/296/dying-with-dignity.pdf (accessed 4.6.15).

Henoch, I., Lövgren, M., Wilde-Larsson, B. and Tishelman, C. (2011) 'Perception of quality of life: Comparison of the views of patients with lung cancer and their family members', *Journal of Clinical Nursing*, 21: 585–94.

Johnsen, A.T., Petersen, M.A., Pedersen, L. and Groenvold, M. (2009) 'Symptoms and problems in a nationally representative sample of advanced cancer patients', *Palliative Medicine*, 23: 491–501.

Johnston, B. and Smith, L.N. (2006) 'Nurses' and patients' perceptions of expert palliative nursing care', *Journal of Advanced Nursing*, 54(6): 700–9.

Kaspers, P.J., Pasman, W., Roeline, H., Onwuteaka-Philipsen, B.D. and Deeg, J.H.D. (2012) 'Changes over a decade in end-of-life care and transfers during the last three months of life: A repeated survey among proxies of deceased older people', *Palliative Medicine*, 27(6): 544–52.

Massie, M.J. (2004) 'Prevalence of depression in patients with cancer', *Oxford Journals,* 32: 57–71.

National Cancer Action Team (2012) *Holistic Needs Assessment for People with Cancer: A Practical Guide for Healthcare Professionals*. London: NCAT. Available at: www.ncsi. org.uk/wp-content/uploads/The_holistic_needs_assessment_for_people_with_cancer_A_ practical_Guide_NCAT.pdf (accessed 4.6.15).

National Cancer Action Team (2015) *A Practical Guide to Holistic Needs Assessment*. London: NCAT. Available at: http://webarchive.nationalarchives.gov.uk/20130513211237/ http://www.ncat.nhs.uk/our-work/living-beyond-cancer/holistic-needs-assessment# (accessed 15.7.2015).

National Comprehensive Cancer Network (2013) *NCCN Distress Thermometer for Patients.* Fort Washington, PA: NCCN. Available at: www.nccn.org/patients/resources/life_with_cancer/pdf/nccn_distress_thermometer.pdf (accessed 4.6.15).

National End of Life Care Programme (2015) *What's Important To Me: A Review of Choice in End of Life Care.* Available at: www.gov.uk/government/uploads/system/uploads/attachment_data/file/407244/CHOICE_REVIEW_FINAL_for_web.pdf (accessed 15.7.2015).

National Health Service (2004) *Improving Supportive and Palliative Care for Adults with Cancer: The Manual.* London: NICE.

National Institute for Health and Care Excellence (2004) *Guidance on Cancer Services Improving Supportive and Palliative Care for Adults with Cancer: The Manual.* London: NICE. Available at: www.nice.org.uk/guidance/csgsp/resources/supportive-and-palliative-care-the-manual-2 (accessed 4.6.15).

National Institute for Health and Care Excellence (2011) *Quality Standard for End of life Care in Adults.* London: NICE. Available at: www.nice.org.uk/guidance/qs13/chapter/quality-statement-5-holistic-support-social-practical-and-emotional (accessed 4.6.15).

Payne, S., Seymour J. and Ingleton, I. (2008) *Palliative Care Nursing Principles and Evidence for Practice*, 2nd edn. Maidenhead: Open University Press.

Pederson, S.N. and Emmers-Sommer, T.M. (2012) '"I'm not trying to be cured, so there's not much he can do for me?": Hospice patients' constructions of hospice holistic care approach in a biomedical culture', *Death Studies*, 36: 419–46.

Sallnow, L., Kumar, S. and Kellehear, A. (2012) *International Perspectives on Public Health and Palliative Care.* London: Routledge.

Stevens, T., Wilde, D., Paz, S., Ahmedzai, S.H., Rawson, A. and Wragg, D. (2003) 'Palliative care research protocols: A special case for ethical review?', *Palliative Medicine*, 17(6): 482–90.

Thomas, K. (2003) *Caring for the Dying at Home: Companions in the Journey.* Abingdon: Radcliffe Medical Press.

Twycross, R. and Wilcock, A. (2001) *Symptom Management in Advanced Cancer*, 3rd edn. Oxen: Routledge.

World Health Organization (2007) *Cancer Control, Knowledge into Action. WHO Guide for Effective Programmes.* Geneva: WHO. Available at: http://whqlibdoc.who.int/publications/2007/9241547345_eng.pdf?ua=1 (accessed 15.7.2015).

World Health Organization (2014) *Global Atlas on Palliative Care at the End of Life.* Geneva: WHO. Available at: www.thewhpca.org/resources/global-atlas-on-end-of-life-care (accessed 15.7.2015).

# 4

# Care planning and changing care needs

## Kersten Hardy and Michelle Brown

---

This chapter will explore:

- the philosophy underpinning care planning
- care planning and how it helps to facilitate the planning and delivery of care
- the patient and their role in the care planning process
- care planning as a platform for discussion
- care planning priority setting
- care planning as a patient reaches the end of life – the complexities.

---

## Care planning philosophy

Care planning is the activity associated with planning care and is an essential part of all nursing interventions; it enables the patient and the nurse to identify their needs and work to specific goals. The ability to complete an effective and thorough care plan with a patient can be affected by a number of variables; experience and knowledge are primary examples. Patients should receive their nursing care from competent healthcare professionals and the patient's dignity should be maintained at all times (NMC 2015). To write an effective care plan, it is important that one understands what it is and how it works in collaboration with physical nursing care (advanced care planning will be addressed in Chapter 9).

# Fundamental aspects of a care plan

A care plan is a document that can either be on paper or in a computerised format and it should be developed in collaboration with the patient (NMC 2015). Care plans may be individualised (produced in response to the specific patient by the nurse undertaking the assessment), core (standardised) or as a pathway to ensure that a patient proceeds along their chosen health journey (Barrett et al. 2012). Although care plans take on different formats, the general principle is to provide details of care needed and a direction and goal for the care delivery. Dorothy Orem (1980, cited by Coldwell Foster and Bennett 2002) recommended that when developing a care plan, one should document the identified problem and the perceived goals in collaboration with the patient. This process requires additional information (e.g. how the goal will be realistically achieved), therefore it needs regular re-evaluation of the patient's progress, with their care plan being reviewed and updated as required. When putting together a care plan it is important to consider that, although as a registered nurse we work concurrently with the standards set by the NMC (2015), we are also responsible for ensuring that the care plans developed are responsive to a number of the standards that apply to direct patient care as developed by the Care Quality Commission (CQC). Primarily these quality outcomes are:

**Outcome 1**: Respecting and involving people who use services. People should be treated with respect, involved in discussions about their care and treatment and able to influence how the service is run.

**Outcome 2**: Consent to care and treatment. Before people are given any examination, care, treatment or support, they should be asked if they agree to it.

**Outcome 3**: Care and welfare of people who use services. People should get safe and appropriate care that meets their needs and supports their rights.

**Outcome 4**: Meeting nutritional needs. Food and drink should meet people's individual dietary needs.

**Outcome 5**: Cooperating with other providers. People should get safe and coordinated care when they move between different services.

**Outcome** : Safeguarding people who use services from abuse. People should be protected from abuse and staff should respect their human rights.

What is apparent from this is that the standards demanded of nurses in the NMC's code of conduct (2015) are echoed here, therefore if we are aware of our responsibilities, patient safety should be maintained and care delivered should be high quality.

> 🗨️   Case scenario: Jacob
>
> Jacob, 46, was diagnosed with motor neurone disease and he has reached the point where communication is difficult and he is struggling to eat and drink. He is under the care of the district nursing team for a pressure ulcer. His mother cares for him and resents anyone coming in to help with care so has refused any help in the past.

## Reflection points

- Apply the quality outcomes identified by the CQC to this case scenario.
- Now map the requirements from *The Code* (NMC 2015).
- How do we ensure that the CQC outcomes and the NMC standards are met?
- Which professionals could help with Jacob's care?
- What do we need to consider before we write his care plan?
- What do we need to discuss with Jacob whilst he can still discuss his wishes?

Jacob is our priority and his wishes need to be determined. In view of his prognosis and likely disease trajectory (difficulties with communication and swallowing), we need to think about the future and make plans with Jacob. A discussion surrounding ethical, legal and end of life issues needs to be undertaken; for example, whether Jacob would want to have cardiopulmonary resuscitation in the event of a cardiac arrest, would he want artificially or clinically assisted nutrition and hydration when he is no longer able to swallow? Patients should have the opportunity to decide what they would or would not want as their condition deteriorates (see Chapters 8 and 9 for further discussion surrounding decision making in palliative and end of life care).

Communication is likely to become more difficult, therefore other strategies to ensure that Jacob can continue to make choices and be empowered for as long as possible should be initiated (e.g. picture boards). Other interprofessional disciplines will need to be involved, so think about his care plan and how it would look. Then think of the professionals who could help to fulfil his care needs in order to achieve the goals (e.g. dietician, specialist palliative care team).

These outcomes essentially reiterate that care planning is patient centred and holistic, that it:

- is developed with the patient and they should be fully included whenever possible
- reflects their need with full consideration being made to their personal choices, culture and diversity.

# The nursing process

Barrett et al. (2012) suggest that a systematic approach to care planning should include the assessment, arrival at a systematic diagnosis, planning, implementing, rechecking (which happens once the documentation of the information has occurred), then evaluating (see Figure 4.1). They suggest this may be more appropriate and reflects the problem-solving requirements a nurse needs to use, rather than the former version of the 'nursing process' (assessment, planning, implementation and evaluation (APIE)). Although they specifically state that the APIE version is not wrong, they felt that the extra elements within this new process emphasise the responsibilities a nurse has regarding their diagnostic reasoning and the recheck as a means of establishing whether the implementation is appropriate (Barrett et al. 2012).

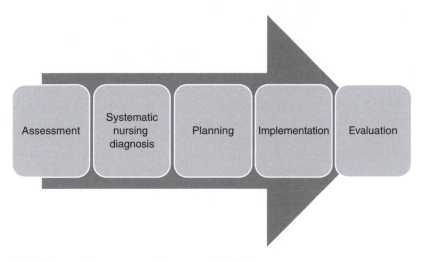

**Figure 4.1**   The nursing process (Barrett et al. 2012)

It is key to emphasise that all aspects of the process remain equally important, with none being more important than the other. Without all elements considered in a robust manner, the care plan may be insufficient or unresponsive to the patients' needs (Lloyd 2010).

# Knowledge and competence

The initial step in developing a care plan is to gather all relevant information from the patient, their family and their medical records. This should incorporate a knowledgeable discussion and enable the patient to express their wishes, fears and concerns. The nurse is required to work with the patient and should perform a holistic assessment (see Chapter 3), ensuring that it remains 'person centred and systematic … and [developed with the patient producing] … a comprehensive personalised plan of nursing care' (NMC 2010: ESC 9.12). The NMC (2010) outlines the importance that proficient care planning has in pre-registration nursing programmes, and so it is vital that one is aware of any deficits in one's knowledge or skill surrounding care planning.

The use of an accredited model of assessment may facilitate the care planning process, but the most important aspect is that it demonstrates that a robust assessment has been performed, including a nursing diagnosis, and that care has been planned based on current evidence (Barrett et al. 2012). The fundamental aspects of care planning are taught to student nurses through a fusion of theory and practice-based learning. The theory element is based on the Roper–Logan–Tierney (RLT) activities of daily living model for nursing (Roper et al. 2000), which is accredited by its use worldwide as a successful framework for all elements of nursing education and care (Holland et al. 2009). Although there are a variety of models available to facilitate the care planning process, such as the Self-care Deficit model by Orem (1959, cited by Coldwell Foster and Bennett 2002) or the Health Care Systems model for nursing developed in 1970 (Neuman 1982, cited by George 2002), the RLT model is the most accepted. It is not uncommon, however, to see in some establishments that to meet their patient's needs or that of the speciality, aspects from a number of models may be used to develop their own method of care plan development (Pearson et al. 2005). The priority is not to focus on which model, but to ensure that patient safety is maintained by operationalising the model(s) in response to patient need, and also that the care planning process is transparent and clear (Barrett et al. 2012). This is essential as care is generally delivered by a team, not one individual, so to ensure that care is seamless and that everyone is working to the same goals or plans, the care plan must be accessible to all members of the team so that everyone involved can follow the plan.

## The Roper–Logan–Tierney model

Within a practice-based environment the basis of nursing care will focus on the same principle of high-quality, safe, patient care, but the documentation and policy may differ from one establishment to another, so it is important to always be aware of the specific policy in your employing Trust. The RLT model refers to the patient's 12 core activities of daily living in both living and nursing models; these provide the structure allowing the development of effective care plans (see Figure 4.2).

It is important to consider when using this model that the patient's goals are realistic in promoting independence and are in concurrence with the patient's coping ability and existing dependency (Pearson et al. 2005). Additional to this process, the development of care plans will help identify any areas where the patient's safety is at risk. Organisations were set up such as the EU Network for Patient Safety and Quality of Care (NHS 2014), which was established three years ago with the intention of bringing together EU members working towards patient safety in healthcare. The aim was to improve patient safety through the sharing of knowledge, expertise and experience, and to improve the quality of care given to patients and their carers.

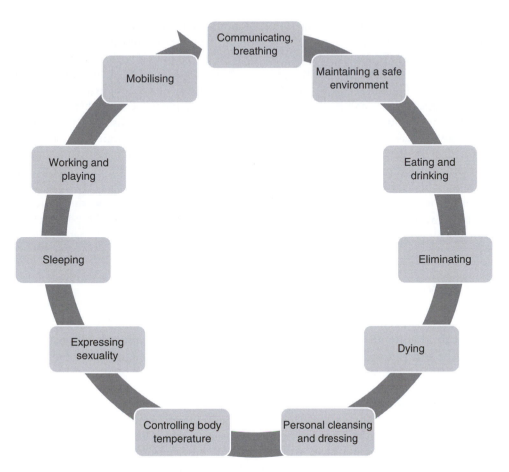

**Figure 4.2**  The 12 core activities of daily living (Roper et al. 2000)

Once the patient has identified the main problems resulting in their need of health-care input, they may start to discuss other problems that they perceive as lower priority to them or which they may feel are irrelevant to their care. It is important to allow time for this process, but as suggested by Gulanick and Myers (2011), the increasing need of people requiring healthcare support and the increasing restrictions of resources available could have a dramatic effect on this aspect of care, causing the patient to withhold information, which may be detrimental to their care and safety.

## Care planning and the assessment process

As briefly discussed, the basic elements of care planning require the healthcare professional and the patient to discuss the patient's needs, which enables the patient to express their concerns and, in turn, allows the healthcare professional to complete a holistic assessment. The healthcare professional who is most likely to carry out this assessment is the nurse, although there may be a multidisciplinary team approach as other professionals are also likely to have contact with the patient. The primary responsibility of the nursing team will be to assess, plan, deliver and evaluate their care (Gulanick and Myers 2011). The assessment process involved in care planning essentially enables the nurse to make a diagnosis (Gulanick and Myers 2011), work alongside the patient and facilitate realistic goals and timescales. Although the assessment period involves primarily verbal communication, another useful skill is the visual observation of the patient and their physical function in developing appropriate plans and goals. Without this full holistic assessment, the nurse may be at risk of missing essential information resulting in a poorly developed or inappropriate care plan. This could have a significant impact on the patient's journey. Evaluating the care delivered also ensures a direction for the patient and their journey.

## Palliative care planning

The holistic assessment of the patient (discussed in Chapter 3) enables the nurse and patient to identify all presenting problems that should be explored. The priorities should be ordered and stipulated by the patient and possible outcomes considered (NICE 2011; NHS 2011). In adult nursing, care planning outcomes can be met in either a short, intermediate or a long-term process; in palliative care, however, the aim is to address problems that the patient feels are having a significant impact on their quality of life, followed closely by other issues which may be equally important to them. The care plan will need to be reviewed on a regular basis, which is identical to a patient who does not have a diagnosis of a life-limiting condition. What one needs to be mindful of is that as they are approaching the end of life, a patient's condition can change rapidly and communication may become very limited or challenging. As a patient deteriorates and/or they need pharmacotherapy, their cognitive function could deteriorate and consequently, their ability to vocalise or express their wishes may be affected. The interprofessional team may be involved in the care planning process as patient issues or symptoms may become more complex (NICE 2011), so clear communication strategies should be employed in addition to clear, unambiguous care plans.

## Reflection point

- Think about what you already understand about care planning, read Mary's case scenario below and identify the areas you would need to address in order to develop an effective care plan for the patient.

> ### 👥 Case scenario: Mary
>
> Mary is 72, lives alone and has advanced breast cancer; she has been admitted into hospital following a fall at home. She is confused and agitated; her family report that she is normally independent but can be forgetful. They have noticed over the last couple of weeks that she has been 'saying and doing some strange things'. Her mouth looks dry, her skin is dry and fragile; she has been incontinent of urine, her clothes and hair look untidy and dirty.
>
> It is clear to see that Mary's condition has changed over a relatively short period of time; she requires care plans that will address her confusion and agitation, dry mouth, dry skin and incontinence of urine. Socially, it is also clear to see that she may have been struggling to manage with her advancing disease. So for each of the identified problems, care plans will need to be written, clearly stating the problem, with documentation of how the problem will be managed, with any investigations appropriate to identify the cause and possible routes of treatment. All medical intervention will be implemented by the medical team and carried out by the nurses where skill remits allow.

The simplistic cause of Mary's deterioration could be a urinary infection, where a course of antibiotics may resolve Mary's symptoms, but additionally this could be a result of her disease process. Complications with the gastro-intestinal system are common in patients with advanced disease and can be caused by the disease itself or as a result of palliative treatment (Hamling 2011). The nurse should develop Mary's care plans by addressing all activities of daily living as she is clearly presenting in such a poorly condition. Mary may feel too ill to contribute to the care planning process, so family and medical notes may assist in this process or an assessment to identify if Mary has the capacity to actively participate, thereby ensuring that Mary's needs are met in the short term. It may be that Mary's condition is reversible and therefore she would be able to contribute at that point. There is also the possibility that Mary is deteriorating, therefore one would hope that advanced care planning has been discussed with Mary at an earlier point in her journey so that her end of life care needs and wishes can be implemented and respected (Brown and Vaughan 2013; Brown 2012; NHS 2011) (see Chapter 9 for further discussion surrounding advanced care planning).

## Challenges to effective care planning

Planning care with a patient who presents with confusion could prove to be a challenge for any healthcare professional. The patient may have a degree of restricted understanding and ability to express their wishes. As acute medical interventions are initiated to help resolve the confusion (e.g. treating an infection or hypocalcaemia), once recovered, the patient may then be able to fully express their wishes.

Patients with dementia, however, may never be able to recover the ability to express their wishes or consent to nursing or medical interventions (Sampson et al. 2010). A randomised controlled trial (RCT) undertaken by Sampson et al. (2010) explored the assessment of patients with dementia who require palliative care. They identified that communication difficulties may present significant obstacles and that carers are reluctant to participate in care planning but are willing to inform healthcare professionals of the patient's history. What should remain important is that patients with a diagnosis of dementia do receive effective palliative care that would meet their personal wishes and goals. Sampson et al. (2010) recommend that this can only be done with advanced care planning. Another significant difficulty that can commonly be encountered in care planning is when a patient presents with a number of extremely complex symptoms and comorbidities, suggesting a need for interprofessional or a variety of specialist support. Seymour and Horne (2013) suggested that many people are now dying with three or more long-term conditions or chronic diseases, therefore the complexities regarding diagnostic reasoning and symptom control may be more prolific as we see this phenomenon increase. The other issue surrounding multiple comorbidities is that with the onset of specialist practice comes a fragmented approach to care of the individual (e.g. a heart specialist, a pulmonary specialist, a gastroenterologist) (Skilbeck and Payne 2003). Even practical aspects like numerous hospital visits to see different specialist teams can be burdensome for patients, and can leave them feeling overwhelmed. The Parliamentary and Health Service Ombudsmen report *Dying without Dignity* (2015) found that there were failures in identifying and linking up people's needs as they approached the end of life and this was more prolific when care was being provided by a number of services, in more than one setting or by more than one provider (Parliamentary and Health Service Ombudsmen 2015). We need to be mindful of these difficulties when planning care and trying to create a holistic approach whereby the patient's journey is seamless and their needs are addressed rather than the specific disease or illness. If specialist teams or other professionals are needed to maximise the quality of care delivered to a patient, then referring the patient to appropriate services may prove beneficial, but we need to ensure that the patient or carer does not feel inundated by the number of professionals who may be involved. Without a cohesive team approach, however, and open communication, the patient may feel that the service is disjointed and haphazard. Consider the following case scenario and think about how you would prepare the care plans.

---

 ## Case scenario: Joe (part 1)

Joe is 88 and has been admitted into your care; he has a diagnosis of cancer of the oesophagus. This is advanced and you can see the tumour pushing tight against his skin on his neck. He has a percutaneous endoscopic gastrostomy (PEG) in situ and is self-caring with this; he uses supplement drinks prescribed by the dietician to maintain his nutritional intake and he gives himself bolus water flushes. His mouth is in poor condition due to tumour intrusion and pain. Joe has uncontrolled pain to the side of his face and neck.

## Reflection point

- Think about Joe's symptoms and what care he will need (e.g. he has pain and will certainly need mouthcare). A patient who is nutritionally compromised may be pre-disposed to a number of other risks; think of these and add them to the care plan.

## Care planning applied to palliative care

First, to try to understand the difference between care planning in general nursing and care planning in palliative care, it is important to remind ourselves about the aims of palliative care. Palliative care is the care of any person that has a life-limiting condition and is no longer related to just cancer. It is the management of symptoms related to an illness in order to promote the quality of life and the prevention of suffering (Cameron-Taylor 2012). It has been referred to as 'end of life care', 'supportive care' and 'hospice care' and has a unique approach to patient care: it is based solely on the quality aspects of living, with the dying process treated as normal and medical care no longer being delivered with a cure-focused route (Cameron-Taylor 2012).

Care planning in palliative care is essentially a similar approach to care planning for a patient who does not have palliative care needs, but requires the healthcare professionals involved to consider that the primary aim is to improve the patient's quality of life, without unnecessary prolonging of life (DH 2008). It is pertinent that the healthcare professional has adequate communication skills, knowledge and understanding of the sensitive issues that will be discussed during the care planning process. For example, a patient who is in the palliative care stage of an illness has already undertaken the first of steps of their journey and has already adapted to a number of changes, primarily to their physical and emotional functioning. These steps are inclusive of diagnosis, treatment and monitoring. The final two steps are disease progression and end of life care, where palliative care is essential in meeting the patient and their loved one's needs as the transitional phase between the final two steps can not only be quick but also prove to be a traumatic and distressing time.

Think again about Joe: his condition has changed whilst he has been in your care, so primarily you would need to refer back to his care plans and revaluate them. It is important and common policy that care plans and risk assessments are updated regularly but also in response to changes in the patient's condition (NMC 2010).

## Case scenario: Joe (part 2)

Joe has been in your care for a week. He is visually weaker on his legs, there is also a small nodule of tumour that is breaking through the skin on his neck and he is spitting out fresh blood. He can still manage to care for his nutritional needs via his PEG, but other members of the team are reporting that he does at times struggle with the feeds and syringes due to his deteriorating dexterity.

## Reflection points

- Would you make changes to Joe's care plan?
- What changes would you make if you decide it needs updating?
- What do you think is happening?
- What should we be discussing?

Joe now needs assistance and his care requires a review. This may include referring back to other members of the multidisciplinary team. Joe may need to be re-assessed by the dietician for increased support in managing his nutritional intake, further discussion with the head and neck specialists and the medical team involved may address Joe's needs regarding the bleeding. This could help to prevent the risk of catastrophic bleed and facilitate a proactive management plan. Joe's disease is progressing, so it would be prudent to have discussions about any specific concerns, so you should discuss his wishes and plan ahead with him.

Patients who have entered the palliative care stage need regular review as their physical, psychological, social and spiritual needs may change rapidly, therefore the care plans should also be updated to address the current requirements. We have identified that care plans should be reviewed with the patient, but consideration must be made to the patient's ability to contribute and make decisions as they deteriorate further. Discussions at an earlier point could help with planning care at this stage, thereby reducing the burden on the patient and their loved ones. If communication is open and realistic, one can plan care in the knowledge that you have some understanding surrounding their wishes as their condition deteriorates (NICE 2011). Goals need to remain realistic and achievable (e.g. to maintain comfort via appropriate pain relief).

Care planning and evaluation should be maintained and continue to involve the interprofessional team. Questioning the planned interventions as the patient's condition deteriorates is essential in ensuring that care remains responsive and appropriate; for example, questioning the appropriateness of physiotherapy input when the patient has entered the terminal phase of life. Let us consider Joe again.

**Case scenario: Joe (part 3)**

Joe has been reviewed by the dietician and has been prescribed a feed that will now be administered via a feeding pump, which no longer requires him to attempt bolus feeds. He is happy for the nurses to complete this intervention for him and to give the bolus water flushes. Joe has been reviewed by the physiotherapist and medical team, and in agreement with Joe and the nurses it has been decided that he will be cared for in bed as he is no longer safe to try to stand due to his overwhelming fatigue.

Sometime later Joe has become unresponsive in his condition and has entered the terminal phase of his life. He requires regular oral care due to the bleeding from the tumour and his medications and feeds are continuing as prescribed via his PEG.

## Reflection point

- Consider how you would react to this situation and document in Joe's care plans any appropriate amendments to ensure that he receives nursing care appropriate to his needs.

For Joe we would need to consider any risks now that he is nursed in bed, so that the care plan can address these.

## Discussing their wishes

The ethical dilemma that surrounds this situation and many others within palliative care can be avoided with the use of advanced care planning. This process refers to a patient's wishes for the future with regard to any medical intervention when they are unable to say what they want. This should be discussed early in the patient's journey and may be initiated by professionals and non-professionals (Burge et al. 2013). Neuberger et al. (2013), who chaired the panel investigating the controversy surrounding the Liverpool Care Pathway, suggested that many of the incidents reported involved poor communication between the medical staff, relatives and carers, which left them lacking understanding and feeling unhappy with the treatment and care their loved ones received. There is a significant barrier to end of life discussions being carried out, as identified by Gott et al. (2009), who noted that GPs rarely discuss the patient's prognosis. This, in turn, may waste valuable time where wishes for the future can be expressed, and result in the patient having no opportunity to discuss his or her end of life care needs. The Parliamentary and Health Service Ombudsman (2015) identified numerous issues surrounding communication at the end of life with patients not being told that they are in the terminal phase of illness, some not even being told a diagnosis, and they suggest that this results in inadequate palliative care in many cases. This dilemma is not rare, as many patients may not wish to know the prognosis early in their diagnosis or the medical professional involved fear they may dash any hope for the patient and family.

The process of end of life care planning or advanced care planning essentially requires excellent communication skills and a trusting relationship. There is no guidance regarding who delivers this information or who has this discussion, but it is often done by nursing teams (e.g. district nurses in the community, Macmillan nurses or specialist nurses) (Bowler et al. 2009). These palliative care skills are important in all areas of nursing. It has been identified that in the community the role of meeting the needs of patients with complex needs is already a challenging one for the community nursing teams. They already facilitate clinical skills, prescribing and end of life care, but it is suggested that their involvement with the patient and developing a relationship of trust before the end of life stage could facilitate conversations regarding end of life wishes (Bowler et al. 2009). Referral to these teams, however, needs to be timely to facilitate the development of the trusting relationship and give time to allow the discussions to take place. A lack of clarity regarding individual wishes can have devastating consequences for both the patient, the carer and the staff involved. As nurses we have an overwhelming need to do the best for our patients, and working without any knowledge of the patient's priorities may lead to feelings of uncertainty and dissatisfaction.

## Nutritional needs at the end of life

Another symptom which can cause distress to family and patients is anorexia. This can complicate the care planning process for a patient with palliative care needs. Raijmakers et al. (2013) identified that patients at the end of life can have a reduced oral intake, with 39–82 per cent of patients receiving palliative care suffering this symptom. It was also one of the highest problematic symptoms resulting in a patient being referred to a palliative care unit in their study. Although we should refer to a dietician and document in the care plan that small but frequent meals be offered, it is important to think about the patient as a whole and address the psychological, spiritual and social needs or issues which may be contributing to the symptom, or how the anorexia may be affecting their quality of life (see discussion in Chapter 10 regarding clinically assisted nutrition and hydration). It is for this reason you are unlikely to complete a nutritional-based care plan that focuses greatly on any weight loss. Watson et al. (2010) have a slightly different perspective as they suggest that patients are not routinely weighed for fear of upsetting them, which may mean healthcare professionals have anxieties about weight loss too. Watson et al. (2010) state that this is acceptable when the patient is in the terminal phase of life only, suggesting that early on in the illness more proactive management may be appropriate as it will enable referral to a dietician, with a positive impact on the quality of life.

It is difficult to plan care with a patient when discussing their nutritional needs; communication skills need to be optimum as it has been identified by Raijmakers et al. (2013) that a reduced appetite can have multiple consequences beyond the actual nutritional value, such as psychological and social pressures. In their study it was identified that a nutritional decline was a notable and significant change to the patient and their relatives. The relatives reported that when the patient was eating and drinking it gave a sense of normality. But the decline in eating and drinking was accepted by some to be the normal process of dying, whilst others felt that the patient had given up the fight against the illness. The results suggest that health-care professionals involved in the assessment process rarely discuss what could be expected and give realistic goals in relation to a patient's reduced appetite.

## Care planning for a patient with a palliative diagnosis versus a non-life-limiting diagnosis

The assessment of need in patients with a palliative diagnosis differs from patients who are not ill with a life-limiting condition. Consider preparing a care plan with a patient who has mobility problems, for example. Patients with cancer or other life-limiting conditions are expected to ultimately decline and their physical function may diminish; this is usually linked with other symptoms related to disease progression. As discussed, nutritional care planning may be complex, and the same applies to a patient's mobility; cachexia, fatigue and psychological withdrawal are pertinent examples suggested by Jordhoy et al. (2007), which complicate the care plan. Being aware of the patient's diagnosis will allow one to consider other possible causes of immobility, such as local manifestations inclusive of spinal cord metastases (cancer that has spread to the spine) and compression (vertebrae that have collapsed and are pressing on the spinal cord resulting in neurological deficits which become irreversible over time) and pathological fractures from bone metastases, especially in the leg/hip area, which would have a significant impact on the mobility of the patient (Jordhoy et al. 2007). Again, the psychological condition of the patient will have a considerable impact on the patient's aptitude to mobilise. This may result in further debility as they fail to improve, which may lead to the perception of being a burden to their family. Feeling a burden is also a significant reason for patients expressing a wish to die, leading to further psychological decline (Jordhoy et al. 2007).

## Conclusion

Comprehensive, individualised assessment of health is necessary to provide the best available planned palliative care (Payne et al. 2008). Additionally, it has been an obvious notation that there is a significant difference between care planning in non-life-limiting illness and those with a palliative diagnosis. Care planning should always take a holistic approach, but this is certainly more obvious in end of life care situations and for those who have a terminal diagnosis, as the complexity of symptoms requires the consideration of psychological, spiritual and social needs as well as physical. In addition, the patient may deteriorate rapidly and to ensure that a proactive approach is taken and that the patient is well prepared for what the journey may hold, an awareness of the disease trajectory and the ability to engage in conversations that can be emotionally demanding can prevent a distressing experience for all concerned.

---

## Sample care plan

Affix Patient Sticker

Care Plan Aim: Palliative/supportive care
Care Plan Goal: To address anxieties and symptoms as needed and to maintain dignity throughout the journey

| Instruction | Date and sign | Review date |
|---|---|---|
| Ensure that the patient understands their condition and is consenting to intervention | | |
| Assess mental capacity as needed when consenting to interventions | | |
| Establish the patient's wishes with regard to resuscitation | | |
| Establish the patient's wishes with regard to hospital admission for reversible conditions | | |
| Liaise with medical practitioner to ensure that the Rightcare Plan is in place | | |
| Identify the patient's PPC | | |
| Discuss the patient's wishes and plan how they can be met | | |
| Review the patient on a regular basis depending on current condition and discuss with the MDT as needed | | |
| Assess the patient's psychological and spiritual needs and implement support as required | | |
| Assess the patient's nutritional and fluid intake and establish alternative options to ensure comfort | | |
| Assess the patient's elimination needs and offer alternatives to reduce anxiety and maintain comfort | | |
| Assess for any symptoms causing distress and liaise with medical practitioner for management methods | | |
| Discuss benefits and burdens of any intervention to allow the patient to make a fully informed decision | | |
| Give the patient sufficient time to express concerns or anxieties | | |
| Implement the end of life care plan according to the patient's preferences when appropriate | | |

**Figure 4.3** Sample care plan

# Suggested reading

Barrett, D., Wilson, B. and Woollands, A. (2012) *Care Planning: A Guide for Nurses*, 2nd edn. Abingdon: Pearson.

Brown, M. (2012) 'Care and compassion at the end of life', *Journal of Care Services Management*, 6(2): 69–73.

National Health Service (2011) *Capacity, Care Planning and Advance Care Planning in Life Limiting Illness: A Guide for Health and Social Care Staff*. Leicester: National End of Life Care Programme.

Neuberger, J., Aaronovitch, D. and Bonser, T. (2013) *More Care, Less Pathway: A Review of the Liverpool Care Pathway*. London: DH.

# References

Barrett, D., Wilson, B. and Woollands, A. (2012) *Care Planning: A Guide for Nurses*. 2nd edn. Abingdon: Pearson.

Bowler, M., Mayne, G. and Gramlin, R. (2009) 'Recognizing the importance of palliative care skills for community matrons', *International Journal of Palliative Nursing*, 15(2): 94–100.

Brown, M. (2012) 'Care and compassion at the end of life', *Journal of Care Services Management*, 6(2): 69–73.

Brown, M. and Vaughan, C. (2013) 'Care at the end of life: How policy and the law support practice', *British Journal of Nursing*, 22(10): 580–3.

Burge, A.T., Lee, A., Nicholes, M., Purcell, S., Miller, B., Norris, N., McArdle, S., Sandilands, S. and Holland, A.E. (2013) 'Advance care planning education in pulmonary rehabilitation: A qualitative study exploring participant perspectives', *Palliative Medicine*, 27(6): 508–15.

Cameron-Taylor, E. (2012) *The Palliative Approach: A Resource for Healthcare Workers*. Cunbria: M&K.

Coldwell Foster, P. and Bennett, A.M. (2002) 'Self-care deficit nursing theory', in J.B. George (ed.), *Nursing Theories: The Base for Professional Nursing Practice*, 5th edn. Upper Saddle River, NJ: Prentice Hall.

Department of Health (2008) *The End of Life Care Strategy*. London: DH.

George, J.B. (2002) *Nursing Theories. The Base for Professional Nursing Practice*, 5th edn. New Jersey, NJ: Prentice Hall.

Gott, M., Gardiner, C., Small, N., Payne, S., Seamark, D., Barnes, S., Halpin, D. and Ruse, C. (2009) 'Barriers to advance care planning in chronic obstructive pulmonary disease', *Palliative Medicine*, 23(7): 642–8.

Gulanick, M. and Myers, L.J. (2011) *Nursing Care Plans Diagnosis, Interventions and Outcomes*, 7th edn. Philadelphia, PA: Elsevier Mosby.

Hamling, K. (2011) 'The management of nausea and vomiting in advanced cancer', *International Journal of Palliative Nursing*, 17(7): 321–7.

Holland, K., Jenkins, J., Soloman, J. and Whittam, S. (2009) *Applying the Roper, Logan, Tierney Model in Practice*, 2nd edn. Philadelphia, PA: Churchill Livingstone Elsevier.

Jordhoy, S.M., Ringdal, G.I., Helbosted, J.L., Oldervoll, L., Havard Loge, J. and Kaasa, S. (2007) 'Assessing physical functioning: A systematic review of quality life measures developed for use in palliative care', *Palliative Medicine*, 21(8): 673–82.

Lloyd, M. (2010) *A Practical Guide to Care Planning in Health and Social Care*. Maidenhead: Open University Press.

National Health Service (2011) *Capacity, Care Planning and Advance Care Planning in Life Limiting Illness: A Guide for Health and Social Care Staff*. Leicester: National End of Life Care Programme.

National Health Service (2014) *EU Network for Patient Safety and Quality of Care*. London: NHS. Available at: www.england.nhs.uk/ourwork/patientsafety/ (accessed 4.6.15).

National Institute for Health and Care Excellence (2011) *Quality Standard for End of Life Care for Adults*. London: NICE.

Neuberger, J., Aaronovitch, D. and Bonser, T. (2013) *More Care, Less Pathway: A Review of the Liverpool Care Pathway*. London: DH.

Neuman B. (1982) *The Neuman Systems Model*. Norwalk, CT: Appleton-Century-Crofts. Cited by J.B. George (ed.) (2002) *Nursing Theories: The Base for Professional Nursing Practice*, 5th edn. Upper Saddle River, NJ: Prentice Hall.

Nursing and Midwifery Council (2010) *Standards for Pre-registration Education*. London: NMC.

Nursing and Midwifery Council (2015) *The Code: Professional Standards of Practice and Behaviour for Nurses and Midwives*. London: NMC.

Orem, D. (1959) 'Guides for developing curricula for the education of practical nurses', cited in J.B. George (ed.), (2002) *Nursing Theories: The Base for Professional Nursing Practice*. Upper Saddle River, NJ: Prentice Hall.

Orem, D. (1980) *Nursing: Concepts of Practice*. New York: McGraw-Hill.

Parliamentary and Health Service Ombudsman (2015) *Dying without Dignity: Investigations by the Parliamentary and Health Service Ombudsman into Complaints about End of Life Care*. London: Parliamentary and Health Service Ombudsman.

Payne, S., Seymour, J. and Ingleton, C. (2008) *Palliative Care Nursing Principles and Evidence for Practice*, 2nd edn. Maidenhead: Open University Press.

Pearson, A., Vaughan, B. and FitzGerald, M. (2005) *Nursing Models for Practice*, 3rd edn. London: Butterwoth Heinemann.

Raijmakers, N.J.H., Clark, J.B., Zuylen, L. van, Allan, S.G. and Heide, A. van der (2013) 'Bereaved relatives' perspective of the patient's oral intake towards the end of life: A qualitative study', *Palliative Medicine*, 27(7): 655–72

Roper, N., Logan, W.W. and Tierney, A.J. (2000) *The Roper Logan Tierney Model of Nursing*. London: Churchill Livingstone.

Sampson, E.L., Jones, L., Thune-Boyle, C.V.I., Kukkastenvehmas, R., King, M., Leurent, B., Tookman, A. and Blanchard, M.R. (2010) 'Palliative assessment and advance care planning in severe dementia: An exploratory randomized controlled trial of complex intervention', *Palliative Medicine*, 25(3): 197–209.

Seymour, J. and Horne, G. (2013) 'The withdrawal of the Liverpool Care Pathway in England: implications for clinical practice and policy', *International Journal of Palliative Nursing*, 19(8): 369–71.

Skilbeck, J. and Payne, S. (2003) 'Emotional support and the role of the clinical nurse specialist in palliative care', *Journal of Advanced Nursing*, 43(5): 521–30.

Watson, M., Coulter, S., McLoughlin, C., Kelt, S., Wilkinson, P., McPherson, A., Wilson, R. and Eatock, M. (2010) 'Attitudes towards weight and weight assessment in oncology patients: Survey of hospice staff and patients with advanced cancer', *Palliative Medicine*, 25(6): 623–9.

# 5

# Supporting carers and families

---

This chapter will explore:

- the need for care
- how to support carers
- the challenges carers face
- co-working between carers and healthcare professionals.

---

## The need for care

Caring carries an emotional burden that may leave the carer feeling stressed, fearful and guilty. There is a growing realisation that caring for the carer is a priority as they may be the person that facilitates end of life care choices (e.g. preferred place of care (PPC) being delivered in the patients' home) (see Chapter 9 for further discussion) (Davies 2003; Grande et al. 1998). The need for informal carers to take on the caring role will undoubtedly increase as the older population (65 years and above) rises. Frailty increases with age from 10–11% in people over 65 rising to 25–50% in those over 85 years of age (NHS England 2014). This does not mean that everyone over 65 years will need care, but what is evident is that there appears to be a significant number of people living with debilitating conditions and/or life-limiting illness who require a potentially increasing amount of care. This challenge has been recognised globally with the realisation that there will also be a need for expert, end of life care nursing (United States Census Bureau 2008; Anderson and Hussey 2000). A great deal of care is currently provided by friends, family or the patient's spouse, and this provision will also need to rise proportionately.

Despite this growing recognition for expert professional staff, the need for well-supported, knowledgeable, informal care givers must also be considered. Currently, however, evidence suggests that caring may be having a significant impact on the carer's quality of life (DH 2008a; Gaugler et al. 2005; Nijboer et al. 1998; Stroebe et al. 2007; Barrow and Harrison 2005).

If carers were paid for the total number of hours of care they provide, this would be greater than the cost of the National Health Service (Buckner and Yeandle 2007). The Department of Health (2008a) recognised the significant impact carers make to healthcare provision and have stated that carers need caring for, which should incorporate assessing their need for support. Support may take on many guises: social, informational and/or emotional and so on. Carers health should be assessed on a regular basis as maintaining their health may mean maintaining the chosen place of care for the one being cared for. If there is a need for an increasing number of carers to take on the physical, psychological, social and emotional task of caring, then investing in the support mechanisms is essential. Maguire (1985) identified that prolonged exposure to grief and suffering may have negative effects on the wellbeing of the carer. Maintaining carers' health should be a key priority. Carers may feel isolated, vulnerable and unsupported by the professionals around them. There are numerous reasons, which can include: lack of information regarding available resources (including financial, equipment); information being delivered but not understood as a result of the stressful situation they may find themselves in; or the use of jargon by the professional.

## What do carers need to care?

Although the *End of Life Care Strategy* (DH 2008b) identified that carers' needs should be addressed, there remains a paucity of services to support them over lengthy periods of time. In the last days of life, services may well be instigated to facilitate death in the preferred place but that carer may have undertaken weeks, months or even years of caring for their loved one with little or no support (Schultz et al. 2003). This prolonged and lengthy period may be exactly what Maguire (1985) was referring to.

There appears to be a period between curative treatment and the last days of life where a carer may feel lost and isolated. Bridges Support Service in the Birmingham area was highlighted in the *End of Life Care Strategy* as a beacon for supporting carers (DH 2008b). There was a recognition in the study from the participants that support needs may take on very different forms, from psychological support to the practicalities of caring or financial advice. If a comprehensive supportive approach is adopted, it can have a significant benefit for those who are in the informal caring role, and who may have no one else to turn to for advice. Unfortunately, there is a dearth of these services and a lack of knowledge surrounding how to contact them and obtain help, so many carers will continue to strive to care alone.

Carers often lose contact with friends and family as they have to allocate more of their time to caring. They may need to relinquish other responsibilities and hobbies or even employment to fulfil the role. A YouGov poll commissioned by Carers UK (2015, see also 2014) suggested that 2.3 million adults have terminated their employment to care for a loved one. This equates to 2,315,433 adults in the UK. Many have reduced their normal working hours or needed to undertake paid overtime work to supplement missed working hours and loss of pay due to caring responsibilities. If a carer has to stop working to give care, this could have significant financial burden on them and potentially other family members if they support them. Additionally, if they have to stop working because they can no longer leave their loved one alone, it may be that their social support diminishes too. This may present a significant burden too, not only their physical health but also their emotional, psychological and social wellbeing. These negative experiences are well recognised in the literature and include:

- Social isolation may be significant as reluctance to leave their relative or loved one once away from work may lead to them limiting social contact outside work with anyone other than the person they are caring for.
- Financial worries and stress associated with being at work adding to the burden.
- Guilt associated with having to be at work and leave their loved one alone or with strangers.

Unfortunately, taking on the caring role may not be a choice that is made for all the right reasons, but may be one made out of having limited choices. Feelings of responsibility or guilt may be the motivation or reasoning behind the choices made. The result may be internal conflict with feelings of regret alongside feelings or recognition of responsibility and wanting to do 'the right thing', but the consequences of this withdrawal from their former life is isolation. As already identified, this isolation may be a significant issue for the carer and affect their psychological and physical health.

## Supporting the carer

There is evidence to suggest that over 58 per cent of deaths occur in hospital (DH 2008b) with a subsequent and increasing drive to ensure individuals spend their last days of life in their home environment whether that environment is a nursing home or their own home. The data suggests that this would be the PPC at the end of life (DH 2008b). This is not just a UK phenomenon; internationally, the majority of care in the last year of life appears to be delivered in the patient's own home (Robbins 1998; Palliative Care Australia 1999). Therefore, it may be that only when things become fragmented or at a point where there is difficulty coping, then admission to hospital may be the option of choice for the carer and/or patient.

The caring tasks themselves can create feelings of uncertainty, inadequacy and lack of self-confidence in the carer (Beaver et al. 2000; Harding and Higginson 2003; Rutten et al. 2005). These unmet needs, including support, may compound the feelings of inadequacy and fear of doing the wrong thing. Bee et al. (2008)

conducted a systematic review of the literature examining carers' practical needs (i.e. how to provide physical care, medication regimes and nutritional care). The results demonstrated an overwhelming need, by carers, for information surrounding emotional and practical support with effective, open communication. Singer et al. (2005) examined carers' satisfaction with communication and healthcare professionals' perceptions regarding communicating information to relatives. Although 74 per cent of carers had been given informational support surrounding the disease, 35 per cent of those were generally dissatisfied with the way it had been delivered, the timing of the delivery and the content of the information. There was a range of issues identified suggesting that individual needs should be addressed. The rate, depth and the timing of that delivery needs a comprehensive assessment and an understanding of the needs of the carers and the patients.

The vulnerability of a carer and patient in a home environment without information surrounding aids, medication regimes, financial support and physical care advice in general should not be underestimated. The use of respite care may help to support the carer in order that they can continue to care for their loved one indefinitely. Caring for a patient with a life-limiting illness is, by the nature of the disease, one where second chances to put things right may not be an option. The poor and distressing experiences will continue long after the patient has died, and the carer may bear the scars of guilt and emotional burnout for a prolonged period (Davies 2003).

 ## Case scenario: Janet

Janet is 42 and she has a full-time job working in a bakery. She has a son, Tim, who is 13. They live in Yorkshire and her mother lives in Northumberland. She visits her mum most weekends and fits in caring for her around her work and son's school and social life. She has not heard anything from Tim's father since he was 2 years old, therefore she only has her mother. She has very little time for socialising herself due to her caring commitments. Her mum had treatment for breast cancer. She recovered well from surgery and had a course of chemotherapy. Janet is now starting to worry about her mum's health as she appears to be losing weight and has general aches and pains. Janet asks her mum to come and live with her so that she can care for her. Janet has a brother but he lives in New Zealand and he rarely calls. Her mum agrees to come but only on a temporary basis, therefore leaves all her furniture in the house and does not put it up for sale. Janet shrugs this off and says she knows her mum would do the same for her but whatever she wanted to do was fine.

The move went well and her mum appeared to settle well. After a few days, however, her mum seemed to become increasingly distressed and the pain increased. She refused to eat so Janet took her to the GP. Following further investigations, her mum was diagnosed with advanced breast cancer which had spread to the liver and brain. The outlook was bleak and Janet felt she had no option but to terminate her employment so that she could care for her mum full time.

Tim, however, was struggling to cope but did not feel he could talk to his mum or grandma because he did not want to upset either of them. Janet was struggling to get any financial help and having difficulties getting any resources or support because her mum was not a permanent resident. Janet struggled to keep her mum comfortable and when helping her to move it seemed to cause her pain. Janet felt isolated and overwhelmed as well as very frightened about what the future held for them all.

## Reflection points

- What difficulties do you think Janet is experiencing?
- Why should we be concerned about Janet?
- Identify the types of support needed for all involved.
- What local and national information is there regarding financial support?

Janet is struggling to care for her mother with the resources available to her. Her own needs are unimportant to her; she may feel isolated and unsupported but needs help to care for her mother during this distressing time. If Janet is left to care it may result in physical injury, having to move her mum around without equipment, but it could also result in injury to her mum. Her social and psychological wellbeing is also of concern as she may be worried about her financial state. She still has a growing son to care for, and this may result in feelings of guilt as she is trying to juggle her time between two people who need her and whom she loves very much. Janet and her son have a variety of support needs to help them deal with the stress and anxiety of caring for a loved one as she approaches end of life.

## Carer needs and consequences of caring

As identified earlier, carers possess unique needs and we must assess and identify those individual needs in order to support them and the patient. Barrow and Harrison (2005) examined the general health of individuals who cared for their loved one in their home. They compared this group with those who cared away from home and non-carers. The carers who cared in their own home suffered significantly more psychiatric morbidity, bodily pain and obesity, which have been associated with premature mortality. Those caring away from home still had significantly more psychological issues, bodily pain and obesity than the non-carers. This demonstrates the considerable poor health outcomes for carers especially if it is in their home, therefore one must be mindful. Health promotion is vital in this population to ensure that they themselves do not become the victims of their caring. In addition, there are differences in responses to prolonged caring amongst different ages, with younger carers reporting more distress. Also, although the data suggests that longer hours of physical care are endured by the older generation (>60 years) (Milne et al. 2001; Buckner and Yeandle 2007) they receive less support from palliative care services (Grande et al. 2006), and financial help is more limited than for younger carers (Seymour et al. 2005) and social support is meager (European Federation of Older People 2004). It may be that as people age the social network becomes more limited because friends and relatives may become frail or they themselves become ill, limiting the support they can offer. What is of concern is that the morbidity and mortality of this age group of carers is significantly greater (Gaugler et al. 2005; Nijboer et al. 1998; Stroebe et al. 2007) than that of younger carers, signifying a greater need for ongoing assessment and additional support. In addition to the differences age may make to carer experience, gender and culture may also play a major role in that experience, but this warrants additional investigation as the research, to date, is limited. Until more evidence becomes available, these differences may be compensated for by utilising the comprehensive assessment strategies suggested and building a rapport and trusting, therapeutic relationship with those charged with caring for a loved one.

## Co-working

The co-worker approach advocated by the Department of Health (2008a) has many benefits. It facilitates the recognition of the carer as a team member who is contributing to the care and wellbeing of the ill person. It suggests a partnership, a philosophy of equality between the carer and professional. This may create a greater harmony and sense of feeling valued and supported in what is a very difficult role. This supposes, however, that access to health and social care professionals has been attained. There will usually be disadvantages to most care approaches and despite the best will, carers may not be 'cared for' in this team approach and feel that they are expected to conform and comply and indeed continue on the 'wave' of the caring role until they are 'washed up' and exhausted (Grande et al. 2009). Care and attention to the individual's needs, including heightened listening skills, are needed in order to identify whether such issues are becoming apparent in the caring environment. Once again, what suits one individual or carer will not suit all carers, just as we are taught that patients are individuals and should be respected as such (NMC 2015).

Carers UK is an organisation fighting for carers' health and rights. They work to ensure that carers' contribution to society, often at the expense of their own health and wellbeing, is recognised. A number of changes in legislation have been announced as a direct result of research and the campaigns that Carers UK have launched, which include: new rights to flexible working for carers; protection from discrimination in equality legislation; and new pension rights (Buckner et al. 2011). This should allow more flexibility for those wishing to continue in paid employment. More importantly, it may help to reduce the financial strain for carers. Carers carry an enormous burden and to add financial worries to this may create greater uncertainty regarding the sustainability of caring.

# Help for carers

The Carers Act 2014 (DH 2014), which came into force in April 2015, may help to change the lives of many carers within the UK. Its premise is that every carer has a right to an assessment which should give access to a range of support services. The range of those services may, unfortunately, be limited in some places but identifying people's needs and trying to respond to those needs should be seen as a step in the right direction. The National Health Service has produced a tool to help identify carers' needs (NHS 2015). It is envisaged that further tools to aid commissioners in meeting the needs of carers will be introduced in the near future, which should help all health and social care staff to assess, identify, plan and instigate strategies to allow carers to care in a safe and supportive environment.

# Conclusion

Despite these changes and initiatives in society recognising carers, there remain too many carers' who struggle to cope and lack the support and professional help they need due to the complexities in navigating through health and social care services. Carers' needs and supporting them to maintain their caring role should be a key strategy. Reasons have been identified within this chapter, from an economic perspective, that the National Health Service could not function without informal carers taking on the caring role. The projected, increasing need for informal carers within society, the recognition that caring may lead to carer burnout with associated morbidity and premature mortality risks, the financial strain of terminating employment or forced termination of employment due to caring responsibilities are all being addressed by ensuring that carers are prepared and supported as much as possible for the caring role by rolling out preparation programmes designed to provide information and education for the carer. By changing legislation to ensure that carers can choose whether they wish to continue to work and care, a choice may then be made rather than a decision being forced on them through lack of options. Over the next decade the plan is to ensure that carers are recognised and supported in their contribution to society and to the wellbeing of their loved ones; however, increasing financial constraints may make these plans increasingly tenuous.

# A carer's narrative

Read and reflect. For this there is no need for reflection points, this true account of a daughter's struggle and her mum's journey says everything. Names have been changed to maintain their confidentiality (NMC 2015).

*(Continued)*

*(Continued)*

## My mum, Emily

When I was first asked to write down my thoughts and feelings surrounding the loss of my mother, my first reaction was, 'Yes, I can do that, I'm in an alright place'. However, the truth is somewhat different: I lost mum five months ago and not a day goes by that she is not foremost in my thoughts. Silly little things trigger a gush of emotions, a Shirley Bassey song on the radio, lilac freesias, bread and dripping sandwiches, and more poignantly a phrase coming out of my daughter's mouth which would be much more in keeping coming out of my mum's! I suppose I fit textbook grief – denial, anger, bargaining, depression and acceptance, the cycle goes on, and depending upon some of the triggers I am aware of like the smell of her favourite flowers will depend on whether I still buy them for her. My sister often buys too much milk, just in case mum runs out.

Mum was 82 when she died on 3/10/2014. She had been unwell for some years prior to her death, and suffered with COPD, angina, underactive thyroid and mobility problems. In the last year of her life she was admitted to our local hospital three times with what we believed to be exacerbations of her COPD. This is where the issues begin and I suppose are chicken-and-egg questions. What am I in these situations, daughter or nurse? Of course I am daughter, but the basic beneficent, nurturing and advocacy role of the nurse cannot be removed. I do not want this to be a dig at a profession of which I am part of, or an unprofessional rant. This is, for me, cathartic in nature writing down how I feel and if lessons can be learnt through this, then great.

Mum's health deteriorated from March 2014 markedly; many GP visits, hospital appointments and community matron visits ensued. Mum said she always felt like she was a nuisance to them and that they did not believe what she was saying. She said she felt like a lost cause and was just waiting to die. I have to say that the difficulties she faced were not fictional, and upon visits to 'specialists' in their field, not in communication I hasten to add, I witnessed first-hand the 'you have COPD, we are doing all that we can, you just have to learn to live with it' attitude. After lots of playing the nurse/patient doctor game, mum finally had a scan on her 82nd birthday. Four days after this mum was struggling to breathe and telephoned the GP; the matron attended and informed my sister and I that she had telephoned for an ambulance and that the results of the scan had indicated she had growths in her lungs and abdomen and that the doctors at the hospital were better placed to inform us more.

I remember looking at mum, who was very calm, despite struggling to breathe. She told my sister and me that she knew, knew all along, and was just sad it had taken them so long to believe her. I was distraught and jumped into medical model, 'lets get her to the hospital fast, I can get her there quicker than the ambulance', and that's what we did, we foolishly entered into a 'let's get her better' mode. We arrived at the busy nurse's station and no one gave us eye contact; we waited patiently despite mum struggling to breath and feeling angry with the news we had been given. We were then ushered in to a busy waiting area and asked to wait, no form of assessment having taken place, and I suppose I flipped. I asked for a qualified member of staff to attend to undertake a set of observations and get mum some oxygen. Reflecting on this, I felt at the time that mum was the priority and was not aware of the pressures the nurse may have been under. My assessment was biased, just like any other relative or patient; the nurses were at a desk and in my opinion could see how anxious we were and should have at least undertaken some obs. My sister and I looked at each other, knowingly, 'don't say anything, remain professional, it's not how we would have managed the situation, but keep going, keep it calm for mum', and that's what we did for the next three hours, waiting, waiting, waiting. We had trundled all of mum's medication into a bag and managed her pain relief with what we had – we adhered to the nurses saying that they were waiting for a bed and that they couldn't give mum anything until she had been seen by a doctor and it had been prescribed. Adhering to policy, that's fine. All we wanted to do was scream, we had so many unanswered questions, had been told to rush to the hospital to get answers, only to be told to wait, in an uncomfortable, crowded area, with no privacy.

As I sat in this area I remember talking drivel to mum: silence was room to think, Eastenders chat was about something not real and stopped me focusing on the news every relative dreads. My sister went to purchase coffee from the main foyer – how strange that memories can be so vivid – asked me what I had for tea yesterday and I struggled; however, ask me what mum's last meal was and I can tell you it was tomato soup, fed to her by my sister, four days before she died (I hasten to add, tomato soup is still not on the menu at my house). When she returned a registrar checked mum in and asked what questions we had – well, the obvious! What is her diagnosis, how long has she had it (hearing it from a doctor was like a rite of passage), what is the prognosis and can we see the scans? I suppose looking back none of us were in the right frame of mind (when are you ever?). A bumbled response was given, and I acknowledge that my questioning must have been argumentative (I remember many times as a nurse dealing with relatives who were scared, angry and just wanted clear, concise and honest information. I hope I managed this well, I think I did, but as the saying goes, 'beauty in the eye of the beholder' – I'm sure there's a better analogy, but I think as a nurse, I did my best to communicate effectively).

I have often thought, was I fair to that doctor, would I have felt the same way, no matter what? I truly believe now, after many months and going over the scenarios time and time again in my head and discussing these with my sister, that his communication was poor. I am now sure of this, when I compare his approach to that of the specialist nurse for palliative care, who took time, away from the hustle and bustle, allowed us to ask questions, without a time constraint, and asked mum what she wanted to happen. After mum's previous admission to hospital, mum had vowed never to go back into hospital again as she felt vulnerable, bullied into doing things she did not wish to do, and frightened. These were her feelings and were valid. Her voice, as with so many older patients, we assume we know best (when I say 'we', I mean nurses). My response was to my sister, 'let's take her home, they can get oxygen at home, I don't want to leave her here'. My belief was that we could care for her better than anyone else. My sister, a nurse also and a less bullish character than myself, wanted desperately to support my wishes and those of mum; however, hers was the voice of reason: 'It's a bank holiday, how can we give 24-hour care, ensure adequate pain relief and manage our families and work?' At this time I saw her as obstructive, not on the same page as me; she made me cross and I told her I would do it without her. Of course she had mum's best interest at heart, and mine too.

As a 'doer' I need to do, therefore I struggled with the inflexibility of the hospital setting. A newly qualified nurse told mum she could not have any more pain relief as it wasn't written up, and I agreed in principle; however, my knowledge of pain relief was such that I knew

*(Continued)*

*(Continued)*

mum could have more pain relief and that it would require a doctor to write this up (I was pulled between being respectful of the nursing staff and acting as advocate for my mum), so I engaged the nurse in further discussion and was told that the doctors were very busy and mum would be okay. I was very angry at this and reminded the nurse that pain was what the patient said it was and that mum was dying, how more important can that be. I think this was the first time I really cried, sobbed – I felt helpless that I could not stop mum's pain and realised that I had to play the game to ensure that mum was cared for adequately. I did not want my actions to make her the 'unpopular patient'.

We managed a move to a local hospice as we were led to believe that her time was short; throughout all of this mum agreed to everything, did not moan, was not outwardly angry, just accepting of the situation, a complete contrast to me. I was supposed to be the strong one. The hospice setting was much calmer, although the reality of it being a place to die was scary. Over the next two weeks my sister and I took turns in visiting mum to ensure that she did not have long periods without us. Her pain relief was the best it had been and mum was settled, had resigned herself to this being her last move. I suppose I felt reassured that mum was okay, as okay as we could get her. We made sure she knew she was loved, really loved. Everyone says how much better hospice nurses are, and yes mum was much more settled. I believe this was down to the team, good communication, effective ancillary support, volunteers bringing drinks round. People actually asking a question and waiting for an answer. Mum was a patient with a name, not just a patient with lung cancer. For this I am truly thankful, for the care we all received in the hospice. However, as mum's pain was controlled she was told, during a time when we were not there to support her, that she needed to go home. When my sister and I returned, mum recounted this as 'they are chucking me out, they want my bed'. Again things were happening outside of our control and plans were being made to discharge her within the next few days. Mum was unsettled again, scared, but resigned herself to going home. A package of care was put in place, key safes were drilled to the bungalow, hello, goodbyes were implemented ('hello, goodbyes', mum's take on the help at meal times), oxygen piped in (without portable cylinders ordered, mum was housebound again). My sister and I again plummeted into 'what should we do for the best?'. Mum was adamant she was going home and would be okay; in truth I knew she wouldn't, and did not want her to go back to her bungalow.

Mum's first night alone at her bungalow, we left her in bed at 10pm, phone at her side, pain medication within reach, with plans for us to go round the next morning. During the night she had a nose bleed which mum could not stop, she panicked and used her buzzer to seek help. The feelings of 'we should have known this was going to happen' kicked in, why on earth did we put mum through this? I felt guilty that we had put her through this, to feel alone and frightened. I still regret letting this happen. My sister said we could take it in turns to stay over and that really we had no other choice. I returned to my original thoughts upon diagnosis, that she should be at home with those she loved and who loved her. The decision was easy for me this time: I would move her in with me. I was conscious this was a selfish decision, I wanted her to be with me, and mum agreed. Looking back, I'm not sure she felt she had any choice. She was frail, vulnerable and scared, something she had been for many months. I was worried that in agreeing to do this, I had not only put myself forward, but my family and sister also. I knew how worried my sister was about how we would cope, physically and emotionally. I didn't give this a second thought, I just knew we had to have her with us.

My husband, son and daughter were supportive and things moved quickly, I emptied what was my daughter's play room, which would become mum's room, beds were moved, oxygen piped, commodes and extra equipment were scattered in all downstairs rooms. I think any logical thinking went out of the window and I focused on making sure mum wasn't scared, but maybe I was focused on me not being scared. Mum never told me she was scared – that might have been the relationship I had with her (I was her baby, being the youngest), as she protected me. I know she spoke more openly to my sister about this. I'm not quite sure how I feel about this; sad that she felt she couldn't tell me, but reassured because she probably knew me better than I know myself and wanted things to be okay for me.

My home became mum's home, my sister's and open house to community nurses, district nurses, hospice liaison, GPs, physiotherapists, occupational therapists, pharmacy services, oxygen delivery people and the hello, goodbyes (for the first few days). I knew for me it was the right move, I hope it was for mum. My sister was fabulous and lived as much at mine as her's. My family adapted well, as did the dogs, to the many visitors and miles of pipe work through the living room and 'play room'. My mum's humour was a little dry at times and I vividly remember her asking the GP if she liked her new room, it was the play room, she chuckled. Over the next weeks I was extremely lucky to share some smiles, laughs, cuddles and long hugs whilst watching re-runs of *Keeping Up Appearances*. Despite having all of these people float in and out of my home, I felt very alone, felt like I had to be strong, keep a brave face and above all, fight for a level of care which I felt was appropriate. I use the word 'fight' loosely, as I don't want you to think I was aggressive, at least I hope I wasn't, and if I was I am truly sorry. I felt like I had to ask for everything, different nasal cannula, to a nasal trough in the hope of reducing the nose bleeds, timely reviews, telephone numbers for out of hours. An example was mum's pain had spiked and the matron had said she would visit to administer subcutaneous drugs with the anticipatory drug pack (the just-in-case medicines) we had been sent home with. However, when she arrived, she did not have the needles and they were not contained in the pack. This made me angry and the time delay in accessing the right equipment meant mum was in more pain. I felt helpless and annoyed that if she had been at the hospice, her time waiting for pain relief would have been shorter. Another example was no slippy sheet for moving mum had been sent; after many phone calls one was located and we could move mum safely. I was partly cross with myself, why had I brought mum home without asking for this? Which was I, daughter or nurse? 'Community care' felt a little like a dumping ground – this is how mum had felt, out of site, out of mind, someone else's problem.

I have reflected at length with my sister in relation to our expectations of the care mum received, were our expectations too high? Did we make care delivery more difficult? Were we best placed to offer her care in her last days? As I stand today, no, my expectations were not too high, I would expect everyone to be treated with respect and dignity with a level of care and compassion, which takes commitment and courage at times to deliver. I think at times the fact that we were nurses made the district nurses feel like they were being watched. Even though the last days of mum's life were us just waiting for her to slip away, the level of love

*(Continued)*

*(Continued)*

and gentle care we offered could not, in my opinion, have been given by anybody better than my sister and myself. I feel proud that we had the strength to care for mum, just as she had cared for us all of her life, and hope that she felt the same way.

On Tuesday, 30th September, mum's pain control was very poor and we were advised that a syringe driver would be the next stage; we were told that she may deteriorate quickly from this point. The driver was in place and working by 12.15pm and mum requested some tomato soup, which my sister sat and gave her a few spoons of. She then lay down to sleep, which would be the last time we would have a coherent conversation with her. I wish so much now that I had said my goodbyes; I am sure, as I told her often enough how much I loved her, that she knew, but this was now final, we lost mum emotionally on this day. I was numb, 'well is this it?' Nobody could tell us how long it would be; mum had breakthrough pain which required additional morphine and these periods were excruciating as she was crying, but as she was semi-conscious we could not reassure her like we had done previously. We would walk into her room, check that she was still breathing. It became too difficult for my children and my nieces to see her this way. For the next three days my sister and I were the only family members to enter mum's room, we took it in turns to sleep on the mattress on the floor at the side of her bed, with another on the sofa in the lounge. We set our alarms to turn mum to prevent her skin breaking down. Sadly, I am ashamed to say we failed in this and mum did have a small area on her sacrum which broke down, and needed a dressing applied by the district nurse. I was devastated that despite our care this had happened, that was all mum needed. I would go into mum's room and sit and just stroke her hand, add Vaseline to her lips and kiss her. I know my sister did the same. I am so glad we had each other.

On 3rd October 2014, after being diagnosed with lung cancer and metastasis in her abdomen six weeks prior, mum slipped away in the arms of my sister and me. We were just moving her to a new position at 11.30pm when we both instinctively observed mum's breathing and searched for a pulse; there was none, we spooned her in her bed and stayed with her until she took her last breath. We were together as she would have wanted, but not in this way, she worried what effect our caring for her would have on us and our families. I am sure she slipped away quickly as she didn't want to be a burden to us and wanted us to get on with our lives. She told us she knew we would be okay, we had each other and our families. I never saw her as a burden, I just wanted to care for her. When mum died I was hugging her from behind and my sister tells me that as she took her last breath a little tear ran down her cheek. I did not see this but know she would have been very sad to leave us. All I remember in these last few moments is that the bed was close to the window, so mum could see 'life outside', and as I clambered on the bed, desperate to love her before she left, I caught the curtain and pulled half of it down – looking back, mum would have laughed so hard at this. Part of me was glad that she had gone, free from pain and suffering, but now the hard part began without her.

Informing all the necessary people ensued and my sister and I kept busy, a coping mechanism. What we did find hard was the fact that only the lady from British Telecom and British Gas offered their condolences. All the health-related people said 'thank you, will make a record of that' – just a number, wipe it from the system. Communication is key and the importance of it underestimated; along with mindfulness it is an essential life skill, which some people have and others don't. Is compassion and caring a skill that can be taught? It is definitely a concept that lends itself to debate, and as a nurse educator my belief is that it is innate but can be harnessed and further developed by training. I suppose we learn by our experiences, and my experience of caring for my mum at home at the end of her life has had a profound effect upon me. As with any experience we try to make sense of it, what could I have done differently, did she know how much I loved her, did we ultimately do right by her? These sadly will be unanswered questions, and depending upon whether I have had a good or bad day will depend on my view of the experience I had.

The overarching issue for me was always the lack of timely, thoughtful and respectful communication. There were also issues with lack of support for carers, emotionally, and supplying the essential practical components needed for such situations. I have tried to offer an overview of how I felt and have cried whilst doing this; there are many areas which I may have missed out as these were too painful. I will offer to show my sister this, but it may be too soon for her and she may not want to share her feelings with me, and may find this counterproductive. I hope not, as I love her deeply and see her as my best friend (obviously along with my husband, who would be upset if I said otherwise).

## Suggested reading

Bee, P.E, Barnes, P. and Luker, K.A. (2008) 'A systematic review of informal caregivers' needs in providing home-based end-of-life care to people with cancer', *Journal of Clinical Nursing*, 18: 1379–93.

Davies, H. (2003) 'The emotional load of caring: Care for those for whom there is no cure', in B. Nyatanga and M. Astley-Pepper (ed.), *Hidden Aspects of Palliative Care*. London: Quay Books.

Stroebe, M., Schut, H. and Stroebe, W. (2007) 'Health outcomes of bereavement', *Lancet*, 370: 1960–73.

## References

Anderson, G.F. and Hussey, P.S. (2000) 'Population aging: A comparison among industrialized countries', *Health Affairs*, 19(3): 191–203.

Barrow, S. and Harrison, R.A. (2005) 'Unsung heroes who put their lives at risk? Informal caring, health and neighbourhood attachment', *Journal of Public Health*, 27(3): 292–7.

Beaver, K., Luker, K.A. and Woods, S. (2000) 'Primary care services received during terminal illness', *International Journal of Palliative Nursing*, 6: 220–7.

Bee, P.E., Barnes, P. and Luker, K.A. (2008) 'A systematic review of informal caregivers' needs in providing home-based end-of-life care to people with cancer', *Journal of Clinical Nursing*, 18: 1379–93.

Buckner, L. and Yeandle, S. (2007) *Valuing Carers: Calculating the Value of Carers' Support*. London: Carers UK. Available at: http://circle.leeds.ac.uk/files/2012/08/110512-circle-carers-uk-valuing-carers.pdf (accessed 15.7.2015)

Buckner, L., Yeandle, S. and Carers UK (2011) *Valuing Carers 2011: Calculating the Value of Carers' Support*. London: Carers UK.

Carers UK (2014) *Costs of Caring and Impact of Caring on Work*. London: Carers UK/
Carers UK (2015) *Caring and Family Services Inquiry*. London: Carers UK.
Davies, H. (2003) 'The emotional load of caring: Care for those for whom there is no cure', in B. Nyatanga and M. Astley-Pepper (ed.), *Hidden Aspects of Palliative Care*. London: Quay Books.
Department of Health (2008a) *Carers at the Heart of the 21st Century: Families and Communities*. London: DH.
Department of Health (2008b) *End of Life Care Strategy*. London: DH.
Department of Health (2014) *Care and Support Statutory Guidance*. London: DH.
European Federation of Older People (2004) *Making Palliative Care a Priority Topic on the European Health Agenda and Recommendations for the Development of Palliative Care in Europe*. Graz: EURAG.
Gaugler, J.E., Hanna, N., Linder, J., Given, C.W., Tolber, V. and Katernia R. and Regine, W.F. (2005) 'Cancer care giving and subjective stress: A multi-site, multi-dimensional analysis', *Psycho-Oncology*, 14(9): 771–85.
Grande, G., Addington-Hall, J. and Todd, C. (1998) 'Place of death and access to home care services: Are certain patient groups at a disadvantage?', *Social Science and Medicine*, 47: 565–79.
Grande, G.E., Farquhar, M.C., Barclay, S.I.G. and Todd, C. (2006) 'The influence of patient and carer age in access to palliative care', *Age and Aging*, 35: 267–73.
Grande, G., Stajduhar, K., Aoun S., Toye, C., Funk, L., Addington-Hall, I., Payne, S. and Todd, C. (2009) 'Supporting lay carers in end of life care: Current gaps and future priorities', *Palliative Medicine*, 23: 339–44.
Harding, R. and Higginson, I. (2003) 'What is the best way to help caregivers in cancer and palliative care? A systematic literature review of interventions and their effectiveness', *Palliative Medicine,* 17: 63–74.
Maguire, P. (1985) 'Barriers to psychological care of the dying', *British Medical Journal*, 29: 1711–13.
Milne, A., Hatzidimitriadou, E., Chryssanthropoulou, C. and Owen, T. (2001) *Caring in Later Life: Reviewing the Role of Older Carers*. London: Help the Aged.
National Health Service (2015) *Commissioning for Carers: Principles and Resources to Support Effective Commissioning for Adults and Young Carers*. London: NHS.
NHS England (2014) *Actions for End of Life Care: 2014–16*. England: NHS.
Nijboer, C., Templaar, R., Sanderman, R., Triemstra, M., Spruijt, R.J., van den Bos, G.A. (1998) 'Cancer and caregiving: The impact on the caregiver's health', *Psycho-Oncology*, 7: 3–13.
Nursing and Midwifery Council (2015) *The Code: Professional Standards of Practice and Behaviour for Nurses and Midwives*. London: NMC.
Palliative Care Australia (1999) *State of the Nation 1998: Report of the National Census of Palliative Care Services*. Yarraluma: Palliative Care Australia.
Robbins, M. (1998) *Evaluating Palliative Care: Establishing the Evidence Base*. Oxford: Oxford University Press.
Rutten, L., Arora, N., Bakos, A., Aziz, N. and Rowland, J. (2005) 'Information needs and sources of information among cancer patients: A systematic review of the research (1983–2003)', *Patient Education and Counseling*, 57: 250–61.
Schultz, R., Mendelsohn, A.B., Haley, W.E., Mahoney, D., Allen, R.S., Zhang, S., Thompson, L. and Belle, S.H. (2003) 'End-of-life care and the effects of bereavement on family caregivers of persons with dementia', *New England Journal of Medicine*, 349: 1936–42.

Seymour, J.E., Witherspoon, R., Gott, M., Ross, H. and Payne, S. (2005) *End of Life Care: Promoting Comfort, Choice and Wellbeing among Older People Facing Death*. Bristol: Policy Press.

Singer, Y., Bachner, Y., Schartzman, P. and Carmel, S. (2005) 'Home-death – the caregiver's experiences', *Journal of Pain and Symptom Management*, 30(1): 70–4.

Stroebe, M., Schut, H. and Stroebe, W. (2007) 'Health outcomes of bereavement', *Lancet*, 370: 1960–73.

United States Census Bureau (2008) *Table 12. Projections of the Population by Age and Sex for the United States: 2010 to 2050*. Washington, DC, US Census Bureau. Available at: www.census.gov/population/projections/data/national/2008/summarytables.html (accessed 4.6.15).

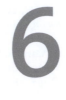

# 6

# Interprofessional working in palliative care

---

This chapter will explore:

- what interprofessional working means
- the qualities needed for effective interprofessional working
- interprofessional working and interprofessional learning
- interprofessional working and policy drivers
- the importance of maintaining effective interprofessional practice for the patient, carer, healthcare professional and organisation.

---

## What is interprofessional working?

Terms like 'interprofessional working', 'interagency working' and 'multidisciplinary working' are often used interchangeably and whilst the underlying principle of working with others remains embedded in all these terms, the core aim should be to work together as a team (interprofessional working) rather than as a number of professionals simply employed in the same setting (multidisciplinary working) (Goodman and Clemow 2008). The Department of Health (2008) stated that supportive relationships should be formed not only between patients and healthcare professionals but also within interprofessional teams to facilitate high-quality palliative and end of life care. There may be a number of professionals actively involved in caring for a patient/service user and their informal carer through their palliative illness, and to ensure they receive the care that is responsive to their specific needs, it requires not only communication and coordination but also teamwork and collaboration to enable this to happen.

'Interprofessional' working denotes professionals working in a collaborative manner. 'Multidisciplinary' does not necessarily denote the collaborative paradigm. Collaboration should be a prerequisite in all care settings, and palliative care is no different. One may argue that as disease progresses, symptoms may become increasingly complex and care management requirements diverse, therefore being able to engage in interprofessional activities should increase the quality and effectiveness of the care delivered (Hall et al. 2006). The principle of having numerous professions in the health and social care setting is to ensure that there is expertise in those settings and a sharing of skills and experience. Without that understanding and 'blurring' of those professional boundaries, care may be fragmented with little understanding amongst professionals surrounding their role and underpinning philosophy. As a registered nurse, the requirement to work collaboratively with other professionals becomes a professional responsibility in itself, and their registration may be at risk if that registered nurse fails to acknowledge or abide by this principle (NMC 2015). Ultimately, one who fails to respond to a patient's needs fails to act in accordance with their code of conduct, and one may argue that failure to collaborate with others will have a direct impact on the care their patient receives and this could be detrimental to the patient's or carer's health and wellbeing.

---

### Case scenario: Lisa

Lisa cares for her father, Ralph, who has dementia. Ralph has been deteriorating and now needs full-time care. Lisa is struggling financially as she has had to give up working, but also feels she cannot leave the house. Her father is struggling to function with any of his activities of daily living. He has also become quite unsteady on his feet and he needs help rising from his bed and from a chair, and Lisa feels things are reaching crisis point. She almost fell with him when bathing him the day before. The district nurse calls and she listens to Lisa's concerns.

---

### Reflection points

- What could the consequences be if the district nurse fails to refer to other health and social care professionals?
- Examine *The Code* (NMC 2015); how does the district nurse breach the code if she fails to act on Lisa's concerns?
- What does *The Code* say regarding working with other professionals?
- How may this enhance care delivery?
- Who will benefit from referral to other professionals?
- List the professional that may be involved in Ralph's care and how they could help.

Although, as professionals like the district nurse in this case scenario, we can have a positive impact on the wellbeing of both the patient and informal carer, what we must recognise is that we have limited understanding and expertise in aspects which historically may be in the domains of 'other' professional's responsibilities (e.g. occupational therapist, psychotherapist or dietician). In this case scenario, Ralph and his daughter are at risk and the district nurse has a duty of care to them both. Examine the NMC's code of conduct (2015) in detail and it will help you to identify your responsibilities as a qualified nurse.

## Understanding roles

There has been much conjecture surrounding role identity, skills and knowledge and power and status (Baxter and Brumfitt 2008). With the evolving socialisation of professional roles, professionals have an advocacy to their individual discipline and although encouraged to work effectively in interprofessional teams, they may feel some conflict between the demands encountered in working in that interprofessional environment and the demands and underpinning philosophies of the discipline. Baxter and Brumfitt (2008) conducted in-depth case studies examining staff perceptions surrounding interprofessional working. Many recounted evident role boundaries and ascribed to the notion that these were important for them as professionals to retain their professional identity. Specific knowledge and skill development was also evident within the specific area and specific profession. The professionals did recognise that there is an increasingly evident shifting and blurring of boundaries; however, the participants did not appear to welcome this development. The political agenda (DH 2008) which calls for blurring of boundaries in order to create an integrated approach to patient care may be a slow process if this study is to be generalised.

## Specialist palliative care teams

Specialist palliative care teams have traditionally used a close, interprofessional approach to care. A vast proportion of patients that require specialist palliative care input have complex needs and a lone worker would soon find themselves overwhelmed by the volume and magnitude of issues, symptoms, needs of the patient, their informal carer and family. As the incidence of multiple comorbidities for older patients rises, these complexities may increase for those with non-cancer as well as cancer conditions. The recognition that specialist palliative care does generally consist of a nurse, doctor and social worker as core members has been acknowledged (Firth 2003), but with the utilisation of the wider team, especially with specialist nurses from different fields of practice contributing to patient care, communication and collaboration may be more difficult and challenging. Dharmasena and Forbes (2001) and Skilbeck and Payne (2005) identified that more collaborative working within teams is essential and perhaps supporting specialist nurses in delivering end of life care rather than handing over to specialist palliative care teams may be the answer for future provision. Therefore, as interprofessional working develops and care becomes more complex, core teams will continue to develop. The core team may not all see the patient and their informal carer but may support each other through regular meetings and offer knowledge, skills and expertise in the hope of improving patient care. Skilbeck et al. (2002) identified that if a patient has a non-cancer disease the opportunity to have specialist palliative care diminishes significantly. In their study, only 4 per cent of the referrals made to the palliative care team had a non-cancer diagnosis yet at the end of life the distress and symptom burden may be similar, suggesting they may have similar or the same needs as a patient with a cancer diagnosis (Skilbeck et al. 1998). As suggested earlier, close liaison with specialist teams and specialist palliative care may help to bridge the gap and ensure that all those at the end of life receive responsive, high-quality end of life care.

Effective and supportive interprofessional working derives significant benefits, not only to patient care but also to the supportive network created through close collaborative working and knowledge sharing. By working collaboratively with professionals like these we can be responsive to the needs of those we are caring for. It is imperative, however, that the patient and informal carer remain empowered throughout this process. Taking over and referring to numerous agencies or professionals will not necessarily have positive outcomes. Potential referrals should be discussed fully with the patient and their carer to ensure that they remain central to all decision making. An influx of professionals into a patient's home or being inundated by professionals whilst in hospital may feel daunting and overwhelming. This will not create that seamless and coordinated, responsive environment we are striving for. Patients may already feel overwhelmed by the nature of their diagnosis and the vulnerability they may perceive, therefore an influx of professionals descending on them and asking questions may well create more problems in its attempt to resolve issues.

## The team approach

The World Health Organization (2010) highlighted the global need for collaborative interprofessional teamworking in order to improve the care that patients/service users receive and to ensure that care is efficient and economical in a healthcare environment which is struggling with financial constraints, but responsive to an increasing number of patients with increasingly complex needs (see Figure 6.1).

To be able to work in an interprofessional environment demands some understanding surrounding how to work with other professionals and teams as well as some insight regarding how the team may support each other utilising their valuable skills and knowledge. Education is fundamental in facilitating that understanding.

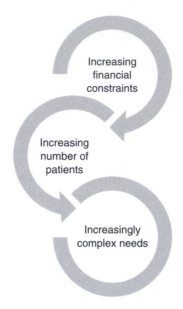

**Figure 6.1**   The current healthcare environment (WHO 2010)

## Education and interprofessional working

The Centre for the Advancement of Interprofessional Education (CAIPE) is an established organisation whose aim is to promote effective interprofessional collaboration and working through education both nationally and internationally (2015). Effective interprofessional education (IPE) can help develop understanding and mutual respect amongst professional groups, and this will have a positive effect not only on patients and their carers/families but also on peers and employers, creating a cohesive and supportive approach to the delivery of patient care. This increased collaboration is the philosophy underpinning health and social care education (Parsell et al. 1998; NMC 2010). The Nursing and Midwifery Council state that an understanding and collaborative approach with other disciplines should be adopted both pre-registration and post-registration (2010, 2015). The Standards of Proficiency which student nurses are assessed against states that knowledge of effective working practices is a requirement and this may be demonstrated through working with other professionals so that they may be familiar with their roles and responsibilities but also how they may work collaboratively with those professionals. One may argue that interprofessional education has been adopted in the academic environment in order to support that learning and foster the team approach whilst breaking down barriers between professionals.

Interprofessional education is more than educating a number of professionals who are sitting together for a lecture; it encompasses learning activities which result in shared learning not only from each other but also about each other. This may be through problem solving or simulation, for example where a sharing of ideas and perspectives can induce greater insight and understanding as well as acknowledging different perspectives surrounding situations or issues. This should facilitate greater understanding and professional respect for each other's contribution in the health and social care environment.

Although interprofessional learning may be facilitated in the academic environment, one may argue that it should be consolidated in practice in order to fully establish interprofessional working into our care provision. Interprofessional working is not only between professionals, however. Students may be allocated a number of environments in which to develop their understanding of health and social care provision and equip them with the skills and knowledge for qualification and entry to the nursing register.

Interprofessional working in practice may be challenging, with team dynamics and the characteristics of the team itself presenting barriers to collaborative working (Hood 2012). Bach and Grant (2009) identified a number of barriers using an adaptation of Arnold and Boggs (2007). They suggested the barriers range from formality of the setting for the interprofessional working to simple issues regarding liking or disliking the person/people within the team. The function of the team and lack of clarity regarding aims and goals can lead to disenchantment and withdrawal (Bach and Grant 2009). In palliative care, having clear goals that have been set by the patient may help to alleviate some of these. As for liking or disliking, professional courtesy and recognising the function of the group – which in this case would be to ensure that a patient has a responsive, caring team to help them through their palliative illness into bereavement – may help to suppress these barriers.

## Patient involvement

Collaboration should take place between professional disciplines, perhaps between private and voluntary sectors but, more importantly, with the patient and informal carer (see Figure 6.2).

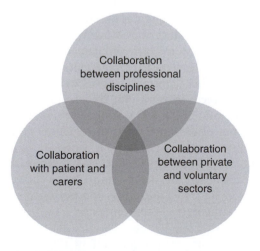

**Figure 6.2** Collaboration in health

Orchard (2010) suggests that interprofessional patient-centred collaborative practice is what we should be striving to achieve, whereby 'the patient retains control over his/her care and is provided access to knowledge and skills of team members to arrive at a realistic team shared plan of care and access to the resources to achieve the plan' (Cook and Hyrkas 2010: 246). The involvement of the patient and carer is essential (see Chapter 5). The palliative and end of life experience may be complex and without the interprofessional approach to care, the physical, psychological, emotional and spiritual needs of the patient and informal carer may not be addressed, resulting in poor care which has been identified as having a 'lasting legacy' for all involved (Cook and Hykras 2010).

## Patients and carers – their contribution to education

Involving the patient and carer in decisions surrounding care planning is paramount, but also has a valuable contribution in the education environment. The NMC (2010) states that user groups are vital in the design and delivery of pre-registration nursing programmes. In addition, they state that they should also have some involvement in the assessment of those students. Turner et al. (2000) have gone further than this and utilised their experience and knowledge in interprofessional education. Patients and carers are acknowledged by the Department of Health (2014) as experts in their condition, but Turner et al.'s particular approach focused on carers' experience in providing care for a loved one at the end of life. A series of workshops was undertaken and facilitated by a palliative care consultant and a lecturer in palliative nursing. Informal carers who were either bereaved or still in the process of caring for their loved one were invited via the hospice to talk about their caring experiences. This provided a novel approach and goes further than the requirements suggested by the NMC (2010). Although simulation has been used extensively in education (Issenberg et al. 2003; Gough et al. 2013; Walsh 2011), this appears to offer a very 'real' approach to education. Students from a variety of interprofessional groups felt privileged to be involved and gained a great deal of understanding and empathy, which can only be a positive experience if transferred to their future practice. Despite the researchers' initial concerns over carer distress and burden, they determined, through focus groups, that the carers felt considerable 'warmth' for the students (Turner et al., 2000: 391). They felt relaxed and at ease in displaying their emotions in front of the students as the students displayed a great deal of maturity, which the carers were surprised about. If we are to suggest that interprofessional working should be patient-centred, then perhaps one may argue that interprofessional education take on that same patient-centred philosophy, involving patients and carers in the education provision not only at the bedside but also in the relative safety of a theoretical environment.

# Common goals amongst the interprofessional team

Health and social care disciplines are bound to codes of practice and conduct that stipulate an expectation that the professional's aim should ultimately be to provide expert, high-quality care to the patient/service user. Building on Firth's suggestions (2003), Sellman (2010) identified requisites for effective interprofessional working: willingness, trust and leadership. Willingness may incorporate not only a willingness to collaborate but also a willingness to recognise each other's contribution and to put others' needs before our own personal needs. Trust is vital for a cohesive approach to patient care. Without a trusting relationship, relying on colleagues for support is diminished and individuals may work in isolation. Leadership, he argues, is vital for the team to function. Having a direction is essential if we are to get anywhere in planning a patient's treatment journey. The values we possess and the ethical stance we take is vital to ensuring that we work and care for each other rather than simply working and caring for ourselves. The reason that we have a number of professionals to work alongside and to work with is because we cannot do everything ourselves. We need to work collaboratively because the human being is a multidimensional individual with distinct and comprehensive needs from a variety of professionals. To understand those professionals, to know that they are there, to be honoured to share and to work with them should be the philosophy we all adopt when interprofessional working is needed.

# Communication

Effective communication is undoubtedly a significant requisite when considering interprofessional working. Barriers to effective communication may present themselves through a variety of situations and issues, from geographical restrictions to the use of profession specific language which presents profession exclusion and may lead to resentment. Communication is the transfer of information or messages using a variety of methods. Enhanced communication may incorporate intended goals or aims of the interaction and involve a conscious and deliberate strategy to achieve the desired goal (e.g. breaking bad news). Breaking bad news involves selecting a model or strategy, and there is a constant checking for understanding and ensuring that it is delivered at a pace which is appropriate for the individual rather than at a pace which is proportional to the appointment slot. Communication does not only occur between the patient and nurse but also between the interprofessional team. Ensuring clarity within the interaction is just as important as that between nurse and patient. Failing to be clear in what one says can be detrimental to another's understanding, and this could result in incorrect care being given as a consequence. We all have a responsibility to reflect on our own communication strategies and acknowledge any weaknesses we may have. Dysfunctional communication is the lack of responsibility or acknowledgement of our communication and leaving the responsibility to others (Smith et al. 2004).

Core conditions for effective communication have been suggested and these include empathy, acceptance and sincerity. Without all these core values and conditions, communication may be at risk of failure due to issues such as misinterpretation and reluctant disclosure as the patient may feel that there is a lack of genuine concern from the healthcare professional leading to a lack of trust.

The effectiveness of the interprofessional team does not only rest upon each other's knowledge surrounding the disciplines: being willing and able to work as a team requires thought and effort. Communication is fundamental to the team's success as well as a mutual respect for each other's opinion and contribution. Goodman and Clemow (2008) debate the differences between a group and a team, emphasising the point that a group of people may work on a ward caring for patients but a team will all work together for the benefit of the patients. Firth (2003) identified that a functioning and effective team needs cohesion and trust, which suggest that merely placing a group of professionals into an environment does not constitute or result in effective interprofessional working. A considered approach is needed and, as suggested earlier, the appreciation of and recognition of each other's values as well as the genuine desire to want work within a team is essential. Incorporating effective and cohesive interprofessional working is not only for our own benefit, but for the benefit of the patient, family, carers peers and the organisation as well.

## Reflection points

- Have you ever felt unable to divulge your anxieties to a friend or colleague?
- Why do you think you felt like this?
- What do you think the difference is between sympathy and empathy?
- Why might empathy be preferable to sympathy?

##  Case scenario: Nigel

Nigel (aged 21) has been diagnosed with testicular cancer. He attends for his first cycle of chemotherapy. The nurse welcomes him to the ward and tries to discuss sensitive issues like hair loss. She gives him information regarding wig fitting. Nigel's partner starts giggling and the nurse feels it is quite inappropriate. Nigel continues through his chemotherapy and the nurse sees the partner laughing again on two occasions when she feels it is inappropriate. She challenges the partner when Nigel has gone for an X-ray. She states that Nigel is very ill and was she aware of this? Nigel's partner becomes very upset. She states that she is well aware of this. Both she and Nigel have always enjoyed each other's company and laughter is how they both get through things. She reveals that she is not sleeping well as she spends all night at home alone, worrying about Nigel and fearing the worst. She thinks that trying to keep things as normal as possible and making him laugh may help to keep his spirits up as this is what he is like, despite the fact that she just wants to break down crying.

## Reflection points

- How do you feel the nurse failed to use the core conditions mentioned above?
- Refer to *The Code* (NMC 2015); what requirements as a registrant did she fail to meet?
- Think about ethical principles; how did the nurse compromise them?
- How could she have supported the couple?
- How would a comprehensive, holistic assessment have prevented this situation?

Judging people is not an activity that is advocated in health and social care. It is really quite the opposite. Recognising people as unique beings with their own set of values and opinions is paramount. This is common to all who work in health and social care. Many working in health and social care have codes of conduct or expected practice to which they must comply (e.g. College of Occupational Therapists, NMC, Health and Care Professions Council, General Medical Council). Patient centeredness, patient empowerment and autonomy are all nouns but more than that, they embody the philosophies underpinning the diverse range of professions which make up health and social care. Ethical principles underpin all care but may become more obvious as one deals with patients who have life-limiting illness. Thinking about the patient's and carer's autonomy, the right to self-determination, especially in a life which is of limited time, beneficence, to do good; caring for Nigel and his partner in the way the nurse did does not fulfil this ethical principle nor that of non-maleficence (to do no harm). One may argue that to challenge Nigel and his partner's coping strategies in favour of ones that the nurse felt more appropriate was highly likely to render the couple distressed, as indeed it did. This leaves the remaining core principle of justice: did the nurse treat the patient and his partner unjustly? These are the four principles – respect for autonomy, non-maleficence, beneficence and justice – suggested by Beauchamp and Childress (2008) and Gillon (1986, 1994). See Chapter 8 for further help regarding ethical principles and ethical dilemmas in practice.

Holistic care allows one to consider the whole person, and if one assumes the same stance when assessing carers and loved ones like Nigel's partner, then they may also be cared for in a compassionate manner. Caring is not simply applied to the patient, but carers and loved ones should also have a degree of consideration for the struggles and anxieties they will also be facing. See Chapter 3 for further help with holistic assessment.

## Reflection points

Think about two separate healthcare experiences where teamwork was very different, either as a nurse or as a patient.

- Was this a positive experience or a negative experience?
- Did they work as a team?
- If they did not, what was missing?
- How could their teamworking be improved?
- How did it feel to work within that team?
- How would you describe the care patients received in these areas?
- How did they communicate with each other?
- What was your perception of staff morale in these areas?

## Teamwork

It may be that you thought of an area that really encompassed all that we have identified regarding effective interprofessional working but may also have identified an area that wasn't so good. The staff morale, patient care, communication and the experience you had of working in the team may have been much more positive in the former rather than the latter. Creating a supportive environment for each other and for our patient is more than just an effective means of providing good care, it also has a positive effect on our working environment, increasing the health and wellbeing of staff and patients. Working as a team takes effort, however, and without everyone contributing one may argue that it can soon be destroyed, and fragmented approaches to care may be adopted with minimal communication between the group involved.

A fragmented approach in palliative care may mean that a symptom or a distressing situation may be unresolved. When a patient has a life-limiting illness, it is not only the individual, but also those around them who may be deeply affected by the situation. There would need to be a professional to lead the interprofessional team to ensure that investigations are not repeated, for example, or questions repeated. The lead would need to cascade any relevant information to the other professionals involved which might need the patient's consent depending on where the information was derived. It also ensures that all members of the team are working to the same aims and goals (i.e. those which have been established by the patient themselves or their loved ones). The holistic care of the patient has been established as paramount in caring for the patient and/or their informal carer/family. Holistic care involves assessing and providing relief and treatment through an understanding of how it may affect the person physically, psychologically, emotionally, spiritually and socially (see Chapter 3). Other members of the interprofessional team may need to be involved in case discussions to help identify how we, as a team, may help the patient/family or informal carer. The team can then identify who should provide the treatment or interventions with the patient's, carer's or family's consent. Without this discussion and collaborative approach, treatment may be biased to the main discipline involved or be narrow and constrained to the resources available to that particular discipline.

 ## Case scenario: Iris (part 1)

Iris is 48 and has been diagnosed with myeloma. She received radical treatment but she has failed to respond. The haematology team is caring for her and are struggling to manage her pain. She seems very distressed at times but the team is unable to deal with the distress. They have had discussions at the team meeting (consultant, junior medical staff and nurse specialist) to try to establish a treatment plan.

A variety of analgesics are prescribed in the hope that one will work. The consultant tries to have a discussion about treatment options with Iris whilst on the ward round but she simply shrugs and suggests that whatever he thinks is best she will do.

## Reflection points

- Why might Iris's pain be unresolved?
- What is the team doing about it?
- What does the team need to do?
- What is happening to Iris whilst the team is developing a treatment plan?
- Who should be involved in the treatment plan?

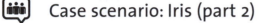 ## Case scenario: Iris (part 2)

The nurses on the ward suggest that the pain Iris suffers may be more comprehensive than purely physical pain. Iris began to chat to the nurse who was providing her personal care, and mentioned that she had lost her daughter a number of years before

*(Continued)*

*(Continued)*

and she wished she was here now. The nurse stopped and decided to sit and listen to Iris. Iris told her of her loss and that it resulted in the breakdown of her marriage, as she could not deal with her death but her husband wanted to move on. She has found it difficult to have any relationships since and has become isolated and estranged from the rest of her family. She now feels worthless and lonely. The nurse asks whether she could discuss her anxiety and distress with the team as they may be able to help her. She agrees and states that she did not feel that this was important or relevant to her current situation. The nurse reassures her and says that they were there to help her even if Iris did not feel that it was relevant to her current condition and situation.

## Reflection points

- What is your understanding surrounding Iris's condition now?
- Which health and social care professionals could help her?
- How should potential referrals be discussed?
- Who makes the decisions?
- How can interprofessional collaboration help Iris?
- What can facilitate effective interprofessional working?
- How will this affect the care that Iris receives?

# Conclusion

Interprofessional working undoubtedly improves patient care, staff knowledge, understanding, support and benefits the organisation. This has been established through clinical data signifying improvement in clinical outcomes and quality of life for those with life-limiting conditions as they approach end of life (NHS 2012). Within the interprofessional team we must recognise that there may be times when members of the team do not agree (Gott et al. 2004), when they perceive conflict between their professional alliance and the team's needs, and when they may feel they are being 'de-professionalised' through the blurring of boundaries. Relationships take work, and relationships exist in the interprofessional team: it is every team member's responsibility to work at improving the interprofessional relationships within the team for the benefit of the patient and their informal carers or family as well as for their own benefit. Interprofessional working requires a willingness to work together, and policy as well as healthcare provision itself demands that of everyone entering the professions. We need to take responsibility but also need to embrace the interprofessional philosophy of all working together as one for the greater good.

## Suggested reading

Cook, M. and Hyrkas, K. (2010) 'Interprofessional team working', *Journal of Nursing Management*, 18: 245–7.

Orchard, C.A. (2010) 'Persistent isolationist or collaborator? The nurse's role in interprofessional collaborative practice', *Journal of Nursing Management*, 18: 248–57.

Skilbeck, J. and Payne, S. (2005) 'Emotional support and the role of the clinical nurse specialist in palliative care', *Journal of Advanced Nursing*, 43(5): 521–30.

## References

Arnold, E. and Boggs, K.U. (2007) *Interprofessional Relationships: Professional Communication Skills for Nurses*, 5th edn. London: Elsevier.

Bach, S. and Grant, A. (2009) *Communication and Interpersonal Skills for Nurses*. Exeter: Learning Matters.

Baxter, S.K. and Brumfitt, S.M. (2008) 'Professional differences in interprofessional working', *Journal of Interprofessional Care*, 22(3): 239–51.

Beauchamp, T.L. and Childress, J.F. (2008) *Principles of Biomedical Ethics*. New York: Oxford University Press.

Centre for Advancement in Interprofessional Education (2015) *Welcome to CAIPE*. Available at: http://caipe.org.uk/ (accessed 4.6.15).

Cook, M. and Hyrkas, K. (2010) 'Interprofessional team working', *Journal of Nursing Management*, 18: 245–7.

Department of Health (2008) *End of Life Care Strategy Promoting High Quality Care for All Adults at the End of Life*. London: DH.

Department of Health (2014) *One Chance to Get it Right: How Health and Care Organisations Should Care for People in the Last Days of their Life*. London: DH.

Dharmasena, H.P. and Forbes, K. (2001) 'Palliative care for patients with non-malignant disease: Will hospital physicians refer?', *Palliative Medicine*, 15: 413–18.

Firth, P. (2003) 'Multi-professional teamwork', in B. Monroe and D. Oliviere (eds), *Patient Participation in Palliative Care: A Voice for the Voiceless*. Oxford: Oxford University Press.

Gillon, R. (1986) *Philosophical Medical Ethics*. Chichester: Wiley.

Gillon, R. (1994) *Principles of Healthcare Ethics*. Chichester: Wiley.

Goodman, B. and Clemow, R. (2008) *Nursing and Working with Other People*. Exeter: Learning Matters.

Gott, M., Seymour, J., Bellamy, G. and Ahmedzai, S. (2004) 'Older people's views about home as a place of care at the end of life', *Palliative Medicine*, 18: 460–70.

Gough, S., Yohannes, A.M., Thomas, C. and Sixsmith, J. (2013) 'Simulation-based education (SBE) within postgraduate emergency on-call physiotherapy in the United Kingdom', *Nurse Education Today*, 33(8): 778–84.

Hall, P., Weaver, L., Fothergill-Bourbonnais, F., Amos, S., Whiting, N., Barnes, P. and Legault, F. (2006) 'Interprofessional education in palliative care: A pilot project using popular literature', *Journal of Interprofessional Care*, 20(1): 51–9.

Hood, R. (2012) 'A critical realist model of complexity for interprofessional working', *Journal of Interprofessional Care*, 26: 12.

Issenberg, S.B., Pringle, S., Harden, R.M., Khogali, S. and Gordon, M.S. (2003) Adoption and integration of simulation-based learning technologies into the curriculum of a UK Undergraduate Education Programme', *Medical Education*, 37(suppl. 1): 42–9.

National Health Service (2012) *Compassion in Practice: Nursing, Midwifery and Care Staff: Our Vision and Strategy*. Available at: www.england.nhs.uk/wp-content/uploads/2012/12/compassion-in-practice.pdf (accessed 4.6.15).

Nursing and Midwifery Council (2010) *Standards for Pre-registration Education*. London: NMC.

Nursing and Midwifery Council (2015) *The Code: Professional Standards of Practice and Behaviour for Nurses and Midwives*. London: NMC.

Orchard, C.A. (2010) 'Persistent isolationist or collaborator? The nurse's role in interprofessional collaborative practice', *Journal of Nursing Management*, 18: 248–57.

Parsell, G., Spalding, R. and Bligh, J. (1998) 'Shared goals, shared learning: Evaluation of a multiprofessional course for undergraduate students', *Medical Education*, 32: 304–11.

Sellman, D. (2010) 'Values and ethics in interprofessional working', in K.C. Pollard, J. Thomas and M. Miers (eds), *Understanding Interprofessional Working in Health and Social Care*. Basingstoke: Palgrave Macmillan, pp. 156–70.

Skilbeck, J., Connor, J., Bath, P., Beech, N., Clark, D., Hughes, P., Douglas, H.R., Halliday, D., Haviland, J., Marples, R., Normand, C., Seymour, J. and Webb, T. (2002) 'A description of the Macmillan Nurse caseload. Part 1: Clinical nurse specialist in palliative care', *Palliative Medicine*, 16(4): 285–96.

Skilbeck, J., Mott, L., Page, H., Smith, D., Hjelmeland-Ahmedzai, S. and Clark, D. (1998) 'Palliative care in chronic obstructive airways disease: a needs assessment', *Palliative Medicine*, 12(4): 245–54.

Skillbeck, J. and Payne, S. (2005) 'Emotional support and the role of the clinical nurse specialist in palliative care', *Journal of Advanced Nursing*, 43(5): 521–30.

Smith, S.F., Duell, D.J. and Martin, B.C. (2004) *Clinical Nursing Skills: Basic to Advanced Skills*. Upper Saddle River, NJ: Prentice Hall.

Turner, P., Sheldon, F., Coles, C., Mountford, B., Hillier, R., Radway, P. and Wee, B. (2000) 'Listening to and learning from the family carer's story: an innovative approach in interprofessional education', *Journal of Interprofessional Care*, 14: 387–95.

Walsh, M. (2011) 'Narrative pedagogy and simulation: Future directions for nursing education', *Nurse Education in Practice*, 11: 216–19.

World Health Organization (2010) *Framework for Action on Interprofessional Education and Collaborative Practice*. Geneva: WHO.

# 7

# Communication in palliative care

---

This chapter will explore:

- the effect good communication can have on patient and carer experience
- strategies that aid good communication
- issues that may hinder communication
- the role communication plays in palliative and end of life care.

---

## Professional responsibilities

Communication is more than a simple dialogue between two or more individuals and, when effective, it can make a huge difference to those involved. It is a complex process as the activity is not simply to relay information, but requires skill and may need specific interventions or aids (e.g. picture boards or an interpreter). The effectiveness of the communication process can be affected by both intrinsic and extrinsic factors, including deficiencies in communication skills. A patient's anxieties about the subject of the communication and the environment in which the communication takes place may have inherent problems, resulting in significant barriers to the communication process. Human beings have a common need: to communicate with those around them. When we nurse a patient, that ability to communicate needs or share information may be hindered by the events leading to their health needs or as a result of other extrinsic or intrinsic issues. What is apparent is that policies and standards emphasise the importance communication plays in ensuring that high-quality care is delivered and, as a result, the positive effect on the patient experience and their general wellbeing (NMC 2010; European Union 2004; DH 2004, 2008; NHS 2003).

The Nursing and Midwifery Council Standards for Pre-registration Nursing Education (NMC 2010) state that graduate nurses need to attain a variety of complex communication skills, whilst respecting the individuality of the person and maintaining their dignity using a compassionate and caring approach. Communication skills are also one of the Essential Skills Clusters, which are specific, minimum standards of competence that have been deemed fundamental at the point of registration (NMC 2007). Once qualified, the nurse remains duty bound to ensure that their communication skills remain effective (NMC 2015).

Communication skills are inherent and underpin all or certainly the majority of NMC standards for pre-registration education (2010). In addition to those identified, the nurse must be able to demonstrate their ability to work as part of a team, and must acknowledge the importance and be capable of interprofessional working. They must be able to delegate, promote health, assess, plan, implement and evaluate care. All these standards require a common skill: communication. To be able to assess a patient, effective communication skills are required: not only to speak clearly and in a tone that is appropriate for the interaction, but to also be able to listen and pick up on non-verbal cues in order to ensure that the interaction has been effective and the patient's assessment holistic. In addition, nurses require interpersonal skills and a degree of self-awareness to ensure that they are perceived as a supportive practitioner who is generally interested and wants to help the individual. A nurse must think about how they intend to approach a patient; how do they intend to communicate with the individual? Have they got any specific needs that may compromise the communication process? When dealing with other members of staff, ensuring the communication event is clear, unambiguous, non-confrontational is paramount for its success. A communication event that goes wrong in this situation may lead to patient harm at its extreme, or risk isolating individuals involved if inappropriate language is used or non-verbal cues indicate an aggressive intent.

## Patient empowerment

Nurse–patient interaction is the most obvious phenomenon where we feel effective communication is paramount. This may incite feelings of anxiety if we perceive the forthcoming interaction as potentially difficult, for example breaking bad news or discussing a very personal matter with the patient. One must remember that effective communication is not as simple as the nurse talking to the patient; it should also involve a great deal of listening too, a nurse can learn a great deal about the patient and their family and this may improve their care experience. Being able to understand a patient's concern is vital when retaining a responsive approach. Facilitating and empowering the patient to identify their priorities is crucial so that we may support them in achieving their aims and goals. Both the National Institute for Health and Care Excellence (2011) and Department of Health (2008) state that patients should feel empowered and central to all decision making, but that in order for them to make the right decision personally, they need to have accurate information delivered in a manner they can understand. To provide accurate information is imperative, and this should include avoidance of technical jargon as this may overwhelm a patient and their loved ones. Using technical jargon has been a significant cause for complaint to the Ombudsman (Parliamentary and Health Service Ombudsman 2014). It may be that the healthcare professionals feel the need to be seen as superior, intelligent or to avoid the impact that the bad news may have on the individual concerned by selecting technical terminology (Witham 2011), but this has an extremely destructive effect. At its worst, the patient may consent to something they do not understand, which, from a legal standpoint, is precarious and involves working outside the law. Patients also have an increased incidence of stress, depression and anxiety when they have experienced significant news broken in a less than adequate manner. It takes a skilled individual to provide information to a patient in a way they understand. Technical or complex situations or procedures require extensive discussion and involve constant checking of the patient's understanding throughout in order to ensure that they are fully informed. All healthcare professionals are duty bound to adhere to this philosophy and approach when dealing with their patients (NHS 2015).

 ## Case scenario: Tracey (part 1)

Tracey has to undergo an examination to investigate the blood in her urine. She receives no information through the post, but is telephoned to ask her to come for an appointment at the outpatient department the following day as they have had a cancellation.

She attends the outpatient clinic and books in at reception. After 10 minutes, a nurse calls her name and asks her to follow. She stops outside a cubicle and asks Tracey to get changed into a gown for her procedure. There should be nothing under the gown and there are some disposable slippers for her to walk over to the treatment room. She does as the nurse asks and is then ushered into a clinical room where a man introduces himself as James.

'Hi, I'm James. Your doctor sent us a letter about your haematuria and said you were concerned.' He does not wait for Tracey to answer and his eyes are fixed on her medical notes where he is perusing the letter. 'We are going to pop a little cystoscope into your bladder and take biopsies. Afterwards you may have some further haematuria and bacterial contamination from the investigation resulting in cystitis. Now pop on the couch, sign your consent form and we will get on with it.' Tracey does as she is asked, signs the consent and lies down as she is instructed. After 10 minutes her investigation is done and she is told to go back to the cubicle, get changed, and she will hear from her doctor.

## Reflection points

- Thinking about the discussion earlier; do you think there are any problems with the consultation?
- What are the ethical and legal implications during this consultation?
- How could it be done better?
- Consider James' approach in the communication process; could this have been improved?

Informed consent is a legal requirement; do you think Tracey was fully informed? Patients undergoing investigations are generally anxious and fear what may be uncovered as a result. Many patients do not know what haematuria is or what a cystoscope is, and 'bacterial contamination' may sound extremely scary. Above all this, Tracey did not have the time to consider the implications of the investigation as she had received no written information and was not given time to receive and process the information that James gave her.

If James had considered his patient as an individual and used his communication skills appropriately, he would have looked at Tracey and potentially seen signs of confusion regarding what he was saying, and signs of anxiety as she was clasping her hands and shaking. In addition he did not ask if she minded that he was male – this is an intimate procedure and some females may feel too embarrassed or self-conscious with a male endoscopist carrying out this procedure.

Let's look at the scenario again, but this time the consultation demonstrates competency in communication and interpersonal skills.

---

### 📣 Case scenario: Tracey (part 2)

After 10 minutes, a nurse calls her name. 'Hello Tracey, I am Ann and I am the healthcare assistant on duty today. I will be looking after you throughout this procedure. Did you receive your information pack?'

Tracey shakes her head and explains that she had received a telephone call the day before. Ann asks her to take a seat on the corridor a moment whilst she speaks to James, 'He will be doing the procedure today, if that is okay with you.' Tracey nods. Ann goes to see James and explains the situation, then escorts Tracey in to see him.

James stands and shakes her hand. He gets her a chair and asks her to tell him why she thinks she is here. Tracey's explanation is brief as she has very little information. James looks at her and suggests that this may all be a little overwhelming. He reassures her and says he will talk to her about the procedure and why it is being performed. Then if she wants to go ahead with it that is fine, and he will get her to sign a consent form after he has explained the risks and benefits, but if she wants time to think about it, that is fine too and he will make her a further appointment for the investigation.

> ## Reflection points
>
> - What is different here?
> - How might Tracey feel?
> - In addition to the improved communication, what other core qualities and skills have the healthcare professionals demonstrated?

Good communication is not just about speaking and giving coherent information. It should encompass the whole process, giving consideration to the patients verbal and non-verbal cues; it should be done in a reassuring, supportive manner so that the patient feels they can share any concerns. It should also ensure that the patient is central to the process, enabling empowerment so that any decisions which may be made as a result of the process are in the patient's best interest. Even asking Tracey to come in to have a discussion before she gets undressed is important, as she may feel more vulnerable wearing just a dressing gown rather than her own clothes.

## The National Health Service Constitution

The NHS Constitution (NHS 2015) equips health service providers and users with guidance relating to what they can expect from their NHS. Its aim is to protect both staff and the public, as well as to provide clarity and give anyone working in the NHS shared goals for service provision and development. The underpinning philosophy of the constitution is person-centred, high-quality care. Good communication has been identified as essential in order to build trust between healthcare providers, including the teams who work together collaboratively, patients and their families. Despite this underpinning philosophy within the former NHS Constitution (2013), poor communication and clinical treatment were the two most cited reasons for complaints about the NHS to the Ombudsman in 2014 (Parliamentary and Health Service Ombudsman 2014). What can be determined from this is that one should never be complacent because the way we communicate to our patients and colleagues matters and can have a significant impact on the way we are perceived and the way the care delivered is perceived.

There are a number of factors that could potentially influence the communication process. The environment, which may be unfamiliar, could be perceived as frightening (e.g. a very clinical environment like intensive care). The individual, who could be either the patient, the healthcare professional or a relative, may affect the effectiveness of the communication process (e.g. conflict or clash of personality). They may not wish to listen to what the other person has to say, or they could have other issues on their mind which limits their concentration. The situation may also have some impact – it may be a difficult discussion which neither the communication sender nor the receiver wants to hear. If it is someone breaking bad news, then previous experience may have an impact on the way the news is received. These examples are not meant to be exhaustive but to give some idea of how messages may be received or sent differently to the intended plan. Therefore one needs to ensure that any messages have been delivered with clarity, that the recipient has a good degree of understanding, and to remember that observation for reactions and body language are crucial throughout the process.

---

 **Case scenario: Ruth**

Dr Smith needs to tell Ruth that her biopsy has come back positive. She hates giving bad news and avoids asking the nurses how she did because she knows that she never handles it well. A nurse accompanies her to Ruth's bedside and to get it over with quickly she tells Ruth 'I am sorry but the biopsy is positive, we will see you in clinic tomorrow to discuss your options now. Erm ... well, the oncologist will be there ... so, erm ... they will have more information for you. I am sorry.' She leaves the room not waiting for Ruth's response.

---

**Reflection points**

- How do you think Dr Smith felt during that consultation?
- How do you think Ruth felt?
- How do you think the nurse accompanying her felt?
- What do you think Dr Smith could do to improve her communication skills?

---

Clearly Dr Smith has significant communication difficulties which affect all those around her. To deliver news like this abruptly and without giving time and space to consider it may have a devastating effect on the patient's journey ahead (Pettifer 2013). Nobody would want to be any of these people in this communication process as it is evident that the process is ineffective, inappropriate and inadequate. Bach and Grant (2011) identify that communication between two or more people where there is a sender and receiver(s) is a process, but this does not indicate the interpersonal element which they suggest is the connectedness between the sender and receiver(s). This is an element which can illicit the caring and compassionate response to people in desperate situations or in overwhelming distress. Without this connectedness the communication, one may argue, would be superficial and inadequate.

## Communicating with those who have a palliative diagnosis

Communication with a patient regarding a cancer diagnosis has been associated with fear and raises questions surrounding one's own mortality (Ferrell and

Coyle 2006). One may argue that any life-limiting illness may invoke such concerns and anxieties. Skilbeck and Payne (2003) suggested that excellent communication is the most important aspect in care provision as this will improve the patient's journey, especially if they are experiencing significant psychological or emotional distress. Dea Moore (2005) suggests that to provide compassionate care at the end of life, healthcare professionals must be able to communicate effectively. Breaking bad news is a responsibility that may present inherent difficulties. Even if the professional possesses advanced communication skills, the patient and their family can present challenges which may adversely affect the encounter, including their previous experiences and expectations about their condition, their caring role and death itself, culminating in death anxiety (Moore 2005; Nicol and Nyatanga 2014). Being responsive and identifying any potential issues or concerns that require addressing is imperative in order to build trust and help the patient and their loved ones through a difficult and distressing journey.

Trice and Prigerson (2009) identified a number of phases which are often associated with a cancer diagnosis, and these may make it easier to discuss and plan for end of life due to this relative predictability. Conversely, the unpredictability of a non-cancer diagnosis may incite difficulties in preparing and discussing end of life wishes. Identifying the 'right time' to discuss deterioration or disease progression may induce great stress for the health professional, but also it may mean that patients and their loved ones are having to think about end of life before they feel that they are approaching the terminal phase. It is difficult to know, however, what is reversible exacerbation of disease and what is end stage, therefore postponing these discussions until it appears more obvious that this is, indeed, the terminal phase of illness, may be too late. What is essential is a very good understanding and experience in dealing with the specific illness involved, as this can help to build up knowledge surrounding indicative symptoms. Ensuring that a holistic assessment is conducted may give a greater understanding surrounding the patient's general quality of life, and a diminishing quality of life may indicate a progressive illness. What is paramount, though, is that the healthcare professional must be assured that their communication skills are sufficient to deal with such discussions.

 ## Case scenario: Alan

Alan suffers with angina and heart failure. He has been experiencing an exacerbation of his symptoms over the last few months. He has required more glyceryl trinitrate to control his angina when walking and has increasingly started to require it at rest. He is experiencing increasing breathlessness and has felt lethargic. He feels disinterested in life as he cannot concentrate on his hobbies and socialising with family and friends has become difficult.

## Reflection points

- How might good communication skills help in this scenario?
- What would your priorities be with Alan?
- Would you be anxious about any specific issues that you feel need discussing?
- Do you think his disease is progressing and, if so, what do you need to do?

It is a difficult time in Alan's journey as he may realise that he is becoming unwell and he will undoubtedly be fearful. Discussing his fears may be what he needs as sometimes the discussion dispels many of the fears, but also understanding what is happening may help Alan to deal with his disease. Sometimes it is fear of the unknown that is difficult to cope with. He may not know who to turn to for help or even know that he should be talking to someone, as his symptoms are a little vague other than his requirement for more glyceryl trinitrate. It is likely that Alan's disease is progressing, and deciding whether one needs to broach the subject of wishes for end of life care is a difficult decision. What is evident here is that Alan has a diminished quality of life, and he may be questioning his purpose and whether life is worth living when feeling as he does. He is socially withdrawing and so may be very isolated, therefore some intervention is needed, and this requires a considered approach where effective communication skills will be essential in ensuring a sensitive interaction where verbal and non-verbal cues are elicited. Alan could feel empowered as a result of his consultation if his fears are addressed and he has the opportunity to discuss his priorities and plan his future care alongside the nurse caring for him.

Being very clear when communicating is obviously essential, but supporting and building a relationship can aid the communication process, as a negative relationship can have a significant adverse effect on any interactions (Moore 2005). Key issues to consider are the environment, ensuring it is as private as possible and comfortable, and not feeling rushed, as the patient and carer may pick up on it and therefore become reluctant to share their concerns or feelings. Having good interpersonal skills and self-awareness are important too, such as active listening skills, facial expressions, body language and an open posture (e.g. not sitting cross-legged with arms folded, as this may inhibit the patient's openness). Thinking about where you will sit and where to sit the patient and their loved ones should be considered, as you need to think that you may need to leave them alone for a little while to digest the information so climbing over people to get out of a room may be difficult. All these sound like logical checks but in a high stress situation forgetting these may hinder the successful outcome of the communication process.

## Good death versus bad death

Preventing distress and supporting through effective communication strategies appear to be causes of great anxiety for healthcare professionals. This may lead to emotion fatigue and burnout (Aycock and Boyle 2009). In addition to the negative effects on the healthcare professional, it can also have devastating effects on the patient and their loved ones, with less than adequate experiences culminating in lack of preparedness as their disease progresses, missed opportunities to discuss their fears and wishes, and more importantly, one may argue that poor communication can be a predisposing factor to a 'bad death'. O'Brien and Jack (2010) identified that poor communication alongside inadequate care planning and coordination results in poorly managed end of life care. Criteria for assisting a good death have been identified and culminate in a desire to express a preferred place of care (PPC), preparedness, spiritual and emotional support, having time to plan and to say what needs saying to those around you (Smith 2000) (see Chapter 10, Death and dying for further discussion). Fisher (2014) identified that communication is central to all nursing activity but becomes more apparent when dealing with those who have a life-limiting illness. To establish a patient's needs requires open dialogue and acceptance, therefore communication plays a fundamental role in achieving the 'good death'. In palliative and end of life care, the situations may be quite complex, requiring patience, acceptance, empathy and sincerity.

 ## Case scenario: David

David was awaiting the results of his biopsy. The doctor entered the room and sat on the chair. David's wife, Melissa, was present. The doctor proceeded to tell them that the cancer had spread. Melissa was shocked and didn't quite understand. She replied, 'You mean he has cancer?' The doctor looked surprised and replied, 'Oh, I thought you knew that already?' He said that David would be seeing the oncologist in a couple of days and then left the room.

## Reflection points

- Could you identify any problems with the way the diagnosis was delivered?
- What was wrong with the doctor's response to Melissa?
- How could this consultation be improved?
- Think of the communication skills used in this scenario.
- What communication strategies could have been employed to improve this consultation?

Breaking bad news is a skill that requires empathy and sincerity and can invoke feelings of apprehension due to fear of upsetting a patient or of not being able to 'handle the situation' (Witham 2011). In this scenario, the doctor here failed to break bad news at a pace appropriate to the patient and their loved one. He did not ascertain their understanding so far. The consequence was a very poor experience for both David and his wife, which could have a devastating effect on their recovery from the news and their future coping strategies (Fallowfield et al. 2002).

## Breaking bad news

This does not always happen as a one-off instance for a patient with a life-limiting illness but may be a series of situations culminating in a wave of bad news. A patient who is on the fifth line of chemotherapy and has been told four times before that it has not worked has bad news delivered on each of those occasions, but the last time may be that 'the disease is progressing despite chemotherapy and therefore we will treat symptoms as they occur now rather than treating the disease'. This may be similar for those with long-term conditions, for example where they have a diagnosis of COPD or multiple sclerosis. They have to face the loss of a life they had, of possible effects to quality and quantity of life, with ultimate consideration of their mortality and what that may hold. The healthcare professional needs to be honest without being brutal in order to facilitate understanding regarding the diagnosis and prognosis, but also to generate feelings of trust (Nicol 2011). This may generate more open communication between everyone involved, and through this open dialogue more support may be generated and perceived. Despite all this, patients may still fear death (Nicol and Nyatanga 2014), but if one can try to allay as many fears as possible and maintain the open dialogue, then gradually this fear may regress.

Breaking bad news should be planned, and having the key facts and understanding surrounding the individual's condition and circumstances may help the healthcare professional deliver this news with some confidence and an empathic tone. Patients and relatives need to have confidence in the skills and understanding of the healthcare professional delivering the news. They need to know that you know what you are doing but also that you care about them as a person, that they are not just one in a very long line of patients you have to see. VandeKieft (2001) introduced the ABCDE model to aid those delivering bad news to deal with it in a planned and progressive manner:

- Advanced preparation
- Building a therapeutic relationship
- Communicating well
- Dealing with patient's and family's reactions
- Encouraging and validating emotions.

This may give the healthcare professional some tangible help at an anxiety provoking time.

# The relationship

Communication between the patient and the nurse relies on the emergence of a therapeutic relationship, therefore a relationship which is deficient of trust and openness may have a detrimental effect on the quality of the communication. A nurse needs to have self-awareness so that they can deal with what may be a demanding palliative care situation, as well as the skills and knowledge to provide the support required (Moore 2005). Non-verbal communication is as imperative as effective verbal communication, and the way the nurse supports the patient can either hinder them in expressing their wishes and fears or help them to feel assured and comfortable in verbalising their concerns (Stajduhar et al. 2010). Stajduhar et al.'s study (2010) examined patients' perceptions of helpful communication. Although the perception may be that supporting a patient and dealing with their anxieties is time consuming, the participants seem to infer that it was not specifically more time that helped improve the support but rather the quality of that time. Direct eye contact and active listening in addition to more obvious aspects like sitting down with the patient rather than standing in front of them, all had a positive effect on the patients' perceptions of supportive communication strategies.

# Professional boundaries

Maintaining professional boundaries does not mean that one should remain detached and emotionally unaffected. Dealing with a patient who is distraught or facing their inevitable demise in the very near future will undoubtedly be challenging and may make the healthcare professional consider their own mortality. Ensuring you feel able to share your anxieties and own personal distress at the situation you are dealing with is paramount in order to continue to care and to cope in the future (see Chapter 11 for further discussion and help). Sharing your emotions and feelings with colleagues you are comfortable with should not be seen as a weakness but actually the opposite: it demonstrates self-awareness and an understanding of the need to debrief in order to protect and care for oneself in order to maintain the level of care and compassion required to deal with all patients in addition to those with a life-limiting illness. Remaining uninvolved and trying to stay emotionally detached may not be sustainable and may result in an emotional detachment that displays itself as uncaring and uninvolved, which is not how a nurse would want to be perceived. Witnessing another human being suffering, if one took a logical approach, is emotive and may make one want to alleviate that suffering. We should consider how we feel about the situation in order to process it (Moore 2005), and sharing that at an appropriate moment is also essential to ensure continued coping with emotive situations, but initially we should consider the patient in order to respond to distress in a timely manner.

## Case scenario: Judy

Judy is a student nurse. She is caring for Alf (aged 55), who has oesophageal cancer and is in the terminal phase of illness. He is upset and she goes over to Alf to ask him what is wrong. He explains that he has not always been a 'good man' and he feels that this cancer is his punishment. Judy is a little overwhelmed and starts to feel upset that this gentleman feels he should be punished. He sees her concern and apologises for sharing this. She holds his hand and shakes her head. 'No I am honoured that you felt you could speak to me. I do not feel that you should be punished at all, but clearly this is something that you have considered and feel, so perhaps we need to help you with this. Would it be possible for me to share this with my mentor so that we could get someone who could talk through your concerns?' Alf agrees.

Judy recounts to her mentor the communication she has had with Alf. Her mentor praises her courage and commitment to care. She suggests the chaplain may help as they are not there only to see those with a specific faith but also to help those who are struggling spiritually and psychologically. Alf agrees to the suggestion and the chaplain spends some time with Alf and this has a positive impact on the way Alf considers his illness and his life. Judy's mentor asks to see her at the end of the shift for a cup of tea. They discuss how Judy handled the situation and talk about how difficult it is to deal with one's own emotions because clearly a patient should not be consoling the nurse but she reassures Judy that yes, he did see she was upset but she did not walk away, she dealt with Alf and his distress in a compassionate, caring manner which has had a very positive result.

Her mentor reassures her that she can come and talk to her at any point if she feels she needs any further help or to talk through things that she may be struggling to deal with. Judy feels reassured and supported. She thinks about the way her mentor helped her and makes a conscious note that she would always try to do the same for any other colleague.

## Reflection points

- How do you think Judy felt when Alf shared his feelings?
- Do you think you could have done what Judy did?
- How do you think you could get support?
- What attributes do you feel the mentor demonstrated?
- How could this have a positive effect on the team?
- How could this have a positive effect on the patient?

Being able to recognise one's own distress is vital, as failure to do so or to ignore it may be unsustainable and result in patients like Alf being neglected and having their concerns unresolved and ignored (see Chapter 11). Effective teamwork does not just mean communicating information but also being able to communicate empathy, compassion and care, which is vital if one wants to be part of a cohesive team. A dysfunctional team may not respond to each other's individual needs, which could leave a team member feeling isolated. If this is left to continue it will grow and soon a number of team members may feel the same. This can result in poor teamwork and have an impact on patient care as a consequence. Staff sickness may ensue, which could be long-term, and this will consequently have a negative impact on the staff left at work, increasing their burden and strain.

## Barriers to communication

Tay et al. (2012) conducted a qualitative study in Singapore and questioned ten qualified nurses working in an oncology unit about perceived barriers to communication with inpatients who have a cancer diagnosis. Amongst a number of barriers identified, which included cultural diversity and the healthcare system challenges, the nurses' own fears were found to inhibit communication, especially when delivering bad news or being unable to answer questions posed by the patient. Difficulties in dealing with emotive situations are not unique to any one culture or geographical area but are far reaching, and may be due to the fact that dealing with human suffering is difficult.

## Communication in palliative care

Open and honest communication is always essential, but in palliative care may involve imparting difficult but highly significant information that could have an impact on the patient's and loved ones' end of life care experience. Communication is often related to disease progression, psychological burden, spiritual wellbeing, social support or symptom management. The participants in Stajduhar et al.'s study (2010) were patients reaching the end of life. They discussed their fear when thinking about a terminal diagnosis, but being able to acknowledge this and to speak about their worries and concerns made the participants more comfortable with the healthcare professional. Sometimes it can just be a case of 'giving permission'. If someone has something that is difficult to speak about, then raising the subject first can help the person to respond and then discuss their concerns. These fears or problems may not be discreet nor easy to deal with; for example, pain may affect a person psychologically as it often represents advancing disease to the patient – it may stop them socialising, it may have an effect on who they are as a person – and there are complexities surrounding the physical presence of pain and trying to alleviate it.

As already established, holistic care should be provided for all patients, but when a patient has a life-limiting illness one may argue that the consequences of the diagnosis alone will be significant; there could also be a cacophony of symptoms that require discussion and assessment in order to try to alleviate the suffering that may ensue. In order for patients to feel that they can discuss their symptoms and their innermost fears, which often go hand in hand, they need to feel that the health-care professional involved really wants to help and is genuinely interested in what they have to say. Any negative feedback they receive, either verbally or non-verbally, could hinder that process. Body language is vital as, although one should not invade a person's space, especially if they are feeling vulnerable, one should not be sat at the other side of the room (i.e. physically distant and formal). Leaning forward slightly may indicate interest in what they are saying and an eagerness to listen. Occasional nodding to indicate understanding with some positive verbal comments (e.g. 'that must be very difficult for you') may help to encourage the patient to continue discussing their concerns.

## Advancing disease

Needs of those who are reaching end of life may include discussions surround-ing advance directives, PPC and preferred place of death (PPD). These can insight a range of emotions for the professional who needs to initiate those discussions (see Chapter 9 for further discussion). Fields et al. (2013) found that nurses working in a hospice feel anxious about discussing PPD, therefore one may suggest that a nurse working in community or acute services may find it more difficult as they may not be as exposed to this type of discussion as a hospice nurse would be.

Dealing with those who have advancing disease demands a compassionate approach, it is a case of not just communicating effectively but delivering informa-tion and help with sensitivity. It is also about openness, and the patient should feel supported, not isolated. Chapters 9 and 10 will deal with end of life care and death and dying in more detail.

## Conclusion

Communication is the basis of all patient and team interaction. Effective communi-cation can make a huge difference to patient and team experience. When dealing with patients who have a diagnosis of a life-limiting illness and their carers, effec-tive, supportive, compassionate approaches to the communication process become even more important as inadequate communication from a professional who feels ill equipped to handle the situation could have devastating effects for all involved, with patients left feeling isolated, angry, misled or confused. Carers may feel helpless in dealing with their loved one and feel dejected with poor experience. This will have a negative impact for any future experiences too.

Healthcare professionals should consider and plan discussions which may be required in order to feel prepared, and to consider the aspects identified in this chapter which can aid the success of the process. They should also reflect on their own performance, seek help where necessary, and ask for feedback to aid improved performance in the future. General openness to patient distress can be informative and rewarding as one can help the patient voice their fears and concerns, which has been reported by patients as being beneficial (Stajduhar et al. 2010).

## Reflection points

- Reflect on your own communication strengths and potential weaknesses.
- In view of what has been covered in this chapter, how do you think you could develop your skills?

## Recommended reading

Parliamentary and Health Service Ombudsman (2014) *Listening and Learning: The Ombudsman's Review of Complaint Handling by the NHS in England 2010–11.* Available at: www.ombudsman.org.uk/healthchp/case-studies2/communication-and-complaint-handling#sthash.dUf36ehU.dpuf (accessed 9.10.14).

National Institute for Health and Care Excellence (2011) *Quality Standard for End of Life Care for Adults.* London: NICE.

Skilbeck, J. and Payne, S. (2003) 'Emotional support and the role of the clinical nurse specialist in palliative care', *Journal of Advanced Nursing*, 43(5): 521–30.

## References

Aycock, N. and Boyle, D. (2009) 'Interventions to manage compassion fatigue in oncology nursing', *Clinical Journal of Oncology Nursing*, 13: 183–91.

Bach, S. and Grant, A. (2011) *Communication and Interpersonal Skills*, 2nd edn. London: Sage.

Department of Health (2004) *Getting Over the Wall: How the NHS is Improving the Patient's Experience.* London: DH.

Department of Health (2008) *End of Life Care Strategy.* London: DH.

European Union (2004) *Enabling Good Health for All: A Reflection Process for a New EU Strategy.* Available at: http://ec.europa.eu/health/ph_overview/Documents/byrne_reflection_en.pdf (accessed 11.6.15).

Fallowfield, L.J., Jenkins, V.A. and Beveridge, H.A. (2002) 'Truth may hurt but deceit hurts more: Communication in palliative care', *Palliative Medicine*, 16: 297–303.

Ferrell, B.R. and Coyle, N. (2006) *Textbook of Palliative Nursing.* Toronto: Oxford University Press.

Fields, A., Finucanel, A. and Oxenham, D. (2013) 'Discussing preferred place of death with patients: Staff experience in a palliative care setting', *British Medical Journal Supportive and Palliative Care*, 3(suppl. 1): A1–A74.

Fisher, J. (2014) 'Communication in palliative and end of life care', in J. Nicol and B. Nyatanga (eds), *Palliative and End of Life Care in Nursing*. Exeter: Learning Matters, pp. 46–64.

Moore, C.D. (2005) 'Communication issues and advance care planning', *Seminars in Oncology Nursing*, 21(1): 11–19.

National Health Service (2013) *The NHS Constitution: The NHS Belongs to Us All*. London: Department of Health.

National Health Service (2015) *The NHS Constitution*. London: Department of Health.

National Institute for Health and Care Excellence (2011) *Quality Standard for End of Life Care for Adults*. London: NICE.

Nicol, J. (2011) *Nursing Adults with Long-Term Conditions*. London: Sage.

Nicol, J. and Nyatanga, B. (2014) *Palliative and End of Life Care in Nursing*. London: Sage.

Nursing and Midwifery Council (2007) *Essential Skills Clusters*. London: NMC.

Nursing and Midwifery Council (2010) *Standards for Pre-registration Nursing Education*. London: NMC.

Nursing and Midwifery Council (2015) *The Code: Professional Standards of Practice and Behaviour for Nurses and Midwives*. London: NMC.

O'Brien, M. and Jack, B. (2010) 'Barriers to dying at home: The impact of poor coordination on community service provision for patients with cancer', *Health and Social Care in the Community*, 18(4): 337–45.

Parliamentary and Health Service Ombudsman (2014) *Listening and Learning: The Ombudsman's Review of Complaint Handling by the NHS in England 2010–11*. Available at: www.ombudsman.org.uk/healthchp/case-studies2/communication-and-complaint-handling#sthash.dUf36ehU.dpuf (accessed 9.10.14).

Pettifer, A. (2013) 'Responding to questions about the end of life', in J. De Souza and A. Pettifer (eds), *End of Life Nursing Care: A Guide for Best Practice*. London: Sage.

Skilbeck, J. and Payne, S. (2003) 'Emotional Support and the role of the clinical nurse specialist in palliative care', *Journal of Advanced Nursing*, 43(5): 521–30.

Smith, R. (2000) 'A good death: An important aim for health services and for us all', *British Medical Journal*, 320: 129–30.

Stajduhar, K.I., Thorne, S.E., McGuinness, L. and Kim-Sing, C. (2010) 'Patients' perceptions of helpful communication in the context of advanced cancer', *Journal Clinical Nursing*, 19: 2039–47.

Tay, L.H., Ang, E. and Hegney, D. (2012) 'Nurses' perceptions of the barriers in effective communication with inpatient cancer adults in Singapore', *Journal of Clinical Nursing*, 21: 2647–58.

Trice, E.D. and Prigerson, H.G. (2009) 'Communication in end-stage cancer: Review of the literature and future research', *Journal of Health Communication: International Perspectives*, 14(suppl. 1): 95–108.

VandeKieft, G.F. (2001) 'Breaking bad news', *American Family Physician*, 64(12): 1975–8.

Witham, G. (2011) 'Communicating with people with long-term health needs', in L. Webb (ed.), *Nursing: Communication Skills in Practice*. Oxford: Oxford University Press, pp. 224–43.

# Dealing with ethical dilemmas

---

This chapter will explore:

- the legal support available to patients with a life-limiting illness
- ethical dilemmas and the application of principles: autonomy; non-maleficence and beneficence; justice; the doctrine of double effect
- the importance of truth and honesty in palliative care
- capacity and its impact on respecting patients' wishes.

---

## Patients' wishes

Ethical issues may present significant dilemmas in healthcare. Some decisions can potentially affect a patient's life, such as withdrawing artificial hydration from a patient at the end of life (Ogston-Tuck 2014). Being able to justify our reasoning is imperative, and understanding ethical principles and our moral obligations to our patients as well as our professional responsibilities can help guide us and ensure that any decisions made have been underpinned by these principles. Within the NMC's code of conduct (2015), there are references to patient empowerment (2.3), respecting a patient's right to accept or refuse care and treatment (2.5), but also recognising and responding with compassion to those who are in the last days and hours of life (3.2). Not only is it a nurse's responsibility to adopt a compassionate approach, to try to maintain patient autonomy and aim to empower the individual in order that they make decisions about what they do or do not want, but also other health and social care professionals have similar professional codes of practice; for example, the College of Occupational Therapists (2011), the Health and Care Professions Council (2012) and the General Medical Council (2013). The right to refuse treatment may incite a great deal of anxiety and concern in the healthcare professional as one needs to feel assured that the patient's decision has been made for the right reason (i.e. because they think their suffering would be far greater if they went ahead with a plan of treatment and not because they feel unworthy of the time spent initiating and administering the treatment/care or because they feel a burden to those around them). Reassuring a patient with a life-limiting illness and trying to establish what they want or do not want and the reasons for those choices may provide a valuable insight into the patient's motivations as well as their anxieties and concerns.

Stanley and Zoloth-Dorfman (2006) suggested that there is an increasing concern that ethical debate, including withholding or withdrawing treatment, what is standard and what is extra-ordinary treatment, and issues surrounding informed consent and truth-telling, is being removed further from patients and those who are mainly affected by these decisions to platforms where they are debated in discussion group settings. Although platforms for ethical debate can help guide us and facilitate the delivery of evidence-based practice, we need to ensure that the patient is treated as a patient with specific needs and that their decisions and autonomy should be respected. Melia (2014) suggests that ethical debate and analysis allow us to determine some context for the relationship between patient and professional and without this the vulnerable (i.e. those reaching the end of life who may feel too exhausted to challenge their care) may, as a result, be at risk of harm. What we need to ensure is that the patient's wishes are clearly articulated by the patient at a time when there are no concerns surrounding the motivation behind the decision, the clarity regarding their capacity to make the decision and, most importantly, before it is too late.

## Autonomy

Autonomy is determined as a positive asset and should be maintained wherever possible as it 'underpins individual liberty and the right that people have to conduct their lives as they see fit' (Melia 2014: 17). Giving a patient the information to be able to make an informed decision about their care should be a fundamental part of our role as a healthcare professional.

 **Case scenario: Bill (part 1)**

Bill was admitted to hospital after suffering a stroke. It affected his ability to swallow, and following the assessment by speech and language therapists it was suggested he remain 'nil by mouth' as he was at risk of aspiration (food and liquid taken orally may go into the lungs rather than the stomach due to a poor gag reflex, leading to infection or pneumonia and potential death). When Bill saw the instructions regarding his feeding requirements above his bed, he became extremely angry and started demanding food.

The doctors and nurses caring for him tried to reason with him, explaining why he was to remain nil by mouth. Despite this he remained adamant that he wanted to be able to eat and drink as he wished.

## Reflection point

- What do we need to do as a team?

It is important for a patient to retain their individual autonomy and be empowered whenever possible. Bill was told about his condition and what the likely outcome would be if he were to eat and drink. The doctors and nurses appear to be working in Bill's best interest according to the Mental Capacity Act (Parliament 2005: s4). In cases like this, it would be important to determine whether Bill has capacity (2005: s2) to make the decision. In addition, it would be worth assessing his psychological state to ensure that he is not depressed, as many patients with long-term conditions (LTCs) have clinically significant depression (DH 2012). This may be due to the duration of the diseases associated with LTCs, which are often protracted, and the affect on quality of life may be significant for the patient (e.g fatigue, dyspnoea and pain).

### Case scenario: Bill (part 2)

A nurse sat with Bill and reassured him that whatever he chose to do, the staff would support his decision, but she wanted to discuss the issues with him. She started by asking him general questions, including his past occupation, who was at home with him and about his stroke. Gradually he began to discuss his feelings about being starved. He had been a prisoner of war and knew what it felt like to be starved. He stated that having been through that once, he was not prepared to go through it again, and, although it may mean that he died as a result, to him it was worth it and it was his choice. She agreed that it was his choice and that he had obviously considered what they were asking him to do. She thanked him and asked if she could share this information with the team caring for him as it would make sense but also because they may be able to give him further treatment. He agreed to this and thanked her for listening to him and for her kindness.

## Reflection points

- How different does Bill's case look now you have the facts?
- Should he be allowed to eat if he wishes?

Listening to patients is crucial when considering any treatment or interventions. What we may wish for ourselves can be completely different to what a patient wishes for themselves. The Mental Capacity Act (Parliament 2005: s1) clearly states that just because we feel a decision is unwise, it does not mean that the person lacks capacity.

Bill has capacity and could fully understand the consequences of eating and drinking therefore, although the staff initially thought his decision was unwise they could not override his decision and assume he lacked capacity. As we progress through this chapter, think of Bill when we address ethical principles.

## Capacity

There are times when a person may be unable to make autonomous decisions and other people may have to consider and treat according to what they feel or perceive is in their best interest. As we can see from Bill's case scenario, this may be quite different to what the patient themselves may, in fact, have wanted. The Mental Capacity Act (Parliament 2005) has given protection to vulnerable individuals and assures them the right to voice their wishes and make choices. If we consider a patient with a life-limiting illness, there could be times when their capacity to make a decision becomes impaired or questionable, such as during acute infection or as a side-effect of opiate analgesia; these examples are potentially reversible, and this should be considered when discussing treatment options and gaining consent. The Mental Capacity Act (Parliament 2005) has allowed us to consider not only whether a patient has the capacity to make decisions, but also to keep in mind their best interests (Dimond 2011). Having the capacity to make one's own autonomous decisions by weighing up the benefits versus harms of treatment may fluctuate, and a patient may have capacity to consent or refuse in some instances but in others they may lack capacity, therefore it is important not to assume a lack of capacity but, quite the contrary, to assume capacity until it has been established otherwise (Parliament 2005: s1, s3). Dimond (2011) refers to this as 'requisite' capacity. It should be assessed for each instance where consent to treatment is required. In end of life care this is particularly apparent when cognitive impairment may have ensued, for a variety of reasons. If, for example, we need the patient to consider whether they would wish to undergo an invasive intervention that may not increase the length of life but may make symptoms a little easier, the disadvantage is that they would require further hospital admission and follow up. The benefits of potential symptomatic relief versus the disadvantages of more time away from home and loved ones for hospital admissions and visits would be better assessed by the patient if they have the capacity to do so. As identified earlier, loss of capacity may be temporary due to an acute presentation which is reversible, therefore every opportunity should be sought to delay consent and decision making until such a time that the causes have been remedied or resolved. In cases where loss of capacity is deemed inevitable and unlikely to be resolved, then discussions should be undertaken with the patient and decisions regarding treatment should be documented whilst the patient can still express their wishes. More formal measures for this may be to develop an advance directive or advance decision to refuse treatment (Parliament 2005: s24). Some patients may feel anxious about advance directives and worry about changing their mind in the future. They should be reassured that it may be revoked at any time, and this can be verbal or written (2005: s24). Patients should therefore be encouraged to think about what they may or may not want as it is important in ascertaining wishes. Other ways that a patient may be able to ensure that decisions are made on their behalf but in line with what they would have wanted would be to appoint a lasting power of attorney (LPA) for personal welfare (Dimond 2011; Parliament 2005: s9).

 Case scenario: Sam (part 1)

Sam, aged 68, had been diagnosed with lung cancer. He had discussed with his sister at great length his wishes for end of life care. He had nominated her as his LPA and documented his wishes with her. Sam was admitted to hospital as his condition had deteriorated significantly. He was confused and distressed. Following blood tests it was determined that he had hypercalcaemia. This was the second time he had suffered with this, so the doctors spoke to his sister. They informed her that it could be treated and he would probably recover but that it would undoubtedly reoccur in the near future. They asked if Sam had considered whether he would want to continue to be treated for this, as there was an option to let nature take its course.

She asked what would happen if he did not have treatment, knowing full well that after his last treatment, once recovered, Sam had said that if it recurred he should be left alone.

The doctors informed her that he would gradually lose consciousness but that it would be important to give some pain relief to ensure that he was comfortable (Watson 2006). His sister refused further treatment on Sam's behalf and asked that he be kept as comfortable as possible.

## Reflection points

- What do you think his sister's motivations are? Consider section 4/5 of the Mental Capacity Act.
- How difficult do you think that decision would be for a nominated LPA?
- What support do you think his sister would need?
- What symptom relief could you give to Sam?
- Think about the core professional ethical principles; what are applicable in this case?

Sam's sister may well doubt her decision, and it would have been one made which held internal conflict for her. She would undoubtedly want her brother to live as she loved him very much and would grieve significantly for his loss. The alternative was that he trusted her to make the right decision for him and to think of his best interest. This carries enormous responsibility and potential suffering during the grieving period (Ogston-Tuck 2014).

## To treat or not to treat

Twycross and Wilcock (2001) state that before treating hypercalcaemia one should consider quality of life prior to the episode and issues such as the frequency or number of episodes of hypercalcaemia. These considerations give those caring for a patient and those with responsibility of LPA a number of facts to bear in mind when deciding on best interests, and treatment withdrawal can only be made on behalf of the patient if they have been deemed to lack capacity (Parliament 2005: s3, s5, s9). If they had a poor quality of life prior to this, perhaps it would be morally right to let nature take its course rather than to prolong suffering, as in Sam's case. The difficulty is that death is inevitable regardless of the decision; note, however, that the patient would need an assessment and have been deemed to lack capacity before the LPA can make any decisions surrounding health and welfare.

## Lasting power of attorney and best interest

Some patients may know that their capacity will inevitably diminish (e.g. dementia). These patients may nominate a LPA. This replaces the enduring power of attorney (EPA), which only applies to property and affairs. The LPA can give the donee (the person nominated by the patient) the power to refuse treatment on their behalf, thereby covering their health and welfare as well as their property and affairs (NHS 2011; Parliament 2005: s4/5) as they will have had the opportunity to discuss this. Their donee can only make decisions about welfare and care if the donor (the patient giving the LPA) has been deemed to lack capacity. That donee should have a clear understanding surrounding any treatments that the donor would refuse. As a result, best interests would be required whereby the LPA would have to give opinion regarding the patient's wishes, and this would be considered as long as they are not making the decision in order to expedite the patient's death (Parliament 2005: s4 (4); Dimond 2011). If the decision was regarding life-sustaining treatment, then the LPA instrument (the written document) would have to be explicit in relation to this. In life-limiting illness it is helpful for the donee to have in-depth discussions with the donor to ensure that they are clear regarding their wishes as such decisions can be overwhelming, and then these should be documented fully and comprehensively to avoid any regret afterwards if there was uncertainty (Khodyakov and Carr 2009).

The Mental Capacity Act stipulates that:

> Where the determination relates to life sustaining treatment he must not, in considering whether the treatment is in the best interests of the person concerned, be motivated by a desire to bring about his death. (Parliament 2005: s. 4/5)

If the patient has not appointed a LPA, then a court-appointed deputy may be employed – referred to as an 'independent mental capacity advocate' (IMCA)

(NHS 2011). They should be instructed and consulted in order to aid decisions surrounding treatment. The difficulty with this is that the IMCA may have very little information, resulting in limited understanding surrounding the patient's own beliefs, values, morals or character in order to work in their best interests. Relatives and friends may be consulted in an attempt to respect the patient's wishes, ensuring every practicable step has been taken to gather information before making decisions on best interests (Parliament 2005, s4 (6), (7); Dimond 2011). Decisions may then be made on the basis of quality of life as perceived by the deputy and distress which may be incurred through prolongation of life with the potential interventions. In cases where the patient is dying from a life-limiting illness, these decisions surrounding prolongation of suffering may be a little clearer as there generally is only further deterioration with little hope of improvement. One can only hope for good symptomatic relief to prevent suffering rather than to aid recovery.

## Non-maleficence and beneficence

As healthcare professionals we are required to uphold the ethical principles, to do no harm (non-maleficence) and only to do good (beneficence). To deprive someone of food may be seen as a breach of one's human rights. If that person is at the end of life and they can no longer eat and drink due to their deteriorating condition, is this depriving them of their human rights? Would it compromise the principle of beneficence to insert an artificial feeding tube, therefore threatening the right to die a dignified and peaceful death? Would this be a deprivation of human rights? One may suggest that it would depend on whether the inability to eat was causing pain or distress. This may be the reason why there is no blanket rule regarding artificial nutrition and hydration at the end of life (such challenges are discussed more fully in Chapter 9).

The case of artificial hydration may take a similar ethical stance: would giving subcutaneous fluids to someone at the end of life be an appropriate intervention? What about the reported pain associated with increased oedema due to the body's inability to control fluid balance (National Council for Palliative Care 2007)? In addition, the NCPC reported that when artificial or clinically assisted hydration was instituted there was an increased incidence of respiratory secretions, urine output resulting in stressing incontinence and diarrhoea which may again contribute to an undignified and potentially distressing death. What artificial hydration can achieve is relief of dry mouth, but think for one moment: are there any other ways to treat a dry mouth than giving artificial hydration with its associated and potential negative effects? Issues surrounding the Liverpool Care Pathway included withdrawal of clinically assisted nutrition and hydration at the end of life (DH 2014). The Department of Health recommended that clear and appropriate discussion takes place with all involved. The Parliamentary Health Services Ombudsman (2015) had complaints surrounding the withdrawal of food and fluids; they ruled that its appropriateness should be assessed on an individual patient basis, that there are times when it may be necessary but conversely times where it may not, and to incur further suffering would be an unacceptable outcome at the end of life.

## Harms versus benefits

Treating symptoms may be a balancing act of harms versus benefits of treatment. As with Sam in the last scenario, to treat would relieve his symptoms, but to what end? In the end stages of lung cancer, patients may be afraid of asphyxia depending on where the tumour is in the lung. Struggling to take one's last breath is understandably a significant fear, therefore giving someone the opportunity to die peacefully and drift into unconsciousness may seem a more ethically and morally desirable goal than intervening with life-sustaining treatments. What is and should be established is whether the patient wishes to undertake life-sustaining treatments. How do we then denote withdrawal of such treatments as ethically and legally acceptable and differentiate this from physician-assisted suicide (PAS), more recently termed assisted dying (AD) (Melia 2014) or euthanasia? Are we not doing the same thing? The difference is that failing to treat a patient who is already at the end of life to die peacefully, rather than to have a death which is likely to involve distress and fear, is not taking action to end a life as in the case of AD or euthanasia. AD and euthanasia involve making a decision and intervening in a proactive manner to end the life of a patient. Mason and Laurie (2011: 565) term it 'therapeutic killing', which is very different from a patient refusing further treatment with the end outcome being the potential for premature mortality. The law is very explicit regarding the active taking of another person's life. Allowing them to refuse treatment which would prolong their suffering involves letting nature and the disease to take its course and not intervening to extend the suffering as in Sam's case scenario above. In addition, healthcare professionals are not obliged to continue to treat someone who is at the end of life if there are no therapeutic or clinical options available (Melia 2014). To treat would extend suffering, which would not be in the patient's best interest, and one may argue is morally and ethically wrong under the principle of beneficence and non-maleficence.

### Reflection points

Think of a patient or patients that you have cared for at the end of life:

- Were they allowed to make decisions?
- If not, what prevented them doing so?
- What could have been done to allow them to make decisions?
- Refer to the core ethical principles and apply them to your patient. Is it a difficult task to do? Are they clear?

Sometimes principles of beneficence and non-maleficence can be difficult to identify and can leave us feeling uncertain of the choices we make. The interprofessional approach to caring for individuals with life-limiting illness can help to ensure that decisions will be made by considering a number of factors as more people may present differing viewpoints, which can be of benefit as long as there can be some resolution. In addition, there may be more support from the team, who may have to help the patient with any difficult decisions.

## The doctrine of double effect

When caring for a patient with a life-limiting illness there may be dilemmas regarding treatments and interventions.

---

 **Case scenario: Harry**

Harry, aged 72, had advanced metastatic prostate cancer, his prognosis was extremely poor and the palliative care team wanted to ensure that he was comfortable as no further treatment was available. He was suffering with significant bone pain, particularly in his hip. He had received radiotherapy to try to treat the pain and the damage to his hip. Opiates had not really helped to relieve his bone pain completely. Although Harry had a history of a past duodenal ulcer, the doctor discussed the possibility of trying a non-sterroidal anti-inflammatory (NSAIDS) as a trial to see if it helped ease the pain (these are a group of drugs which reduce inflammation which is a key factor in the pain associated with bone metastases) but one of the side effects is gastric irritation. This would carry a risk in view of his medical history (i.e. he may develop a gastric or duodenal bleed from the previous ulcer site). Harry knew that time was short and the thought of dying in pain terrified him. He wanted to be free of pain so that he could do the things he wanted to do before he died. He agreed to the treatment.

---

## Reflection point

- Could you apply the doctrine of double effect?

---

Harry had the capacity to make decisions, and although this treatment was a risk to his life it would also give him added quality in the remainder of his life if it eased his pain. He was allowed to practice his autonomy in making decisions about his treatment. Justification for offering the drug treatment was made using the four main ethical principles of respect for autonomy, non-maleficence, beneficence and justice (Beauchamp and Childress 2008). Harry had the capacity to make decisions, and the team wanted only to 'do good', which was to ease his pain (beneficence).

They did not want to leave him in pain, nor to give him a treatment that would be potentially harmful without his full knowledge (non-maleficence). Justice involves being fair, treating people with fairness. Giving Harry the information so that he could make his own decision was to deliver fair treatment.

Melia (2014) suggests that ethics allows us to examine our moral reasoning through moral debate. This should help guide us and provide reassurance as we embark on our caring role every day. We cannot ignore ethics, it is inherent in everything we do, and every decision we make depends on our values, beliefs and morals but we also have to consider our professional and legal requirements. Palliative and end of life care present myriad significant ethical dilemmas, and these may often have life and death considerations. As health and social care professionals we have a responsibility to ensure that patient wellbeing and quality of life are the priority, and to utilise ethical principles and the law to examine and explain our decisions.

## Recommended reading

Beauchamp, T.M. and Childress, J.F. (2008) *Principles of Biomedical Ethics*, 6th edn. Oxford: Oxford University Press.

National Council for Palliative Care (2007) *Artificial Nutrition and Hydration*. London: NCPC.

Parliament (2005) *Mental Capacity Act 2005 Elizabeth II*. London: The Stationary Office. Chapter 9. Available at: www.legislation.gov.uk/ukpga/2005/9/contents (accessed 15.7.2015).

Parliamentary and Health Service Ombudsman (2015) *Dying without Dignity: Investigations by the Parliamentary and Health Service Ombudsman into Complaints about End of Life Care*. London: Parliamentary and Health Service Ombudsman.

## References

Beauchamp, T.M. and Childress, J.F. (2008) *Principles of Biomedical Ethics*, 6th edn. Oxford: Oxford University Press.

College of Occupational Therapists (2011) *Professional Standards for Occupational Therapy Practice*. England: COT.

Department of Health (2012) *Long-Term Conditions Compendium of Information*, 3rd edn. London: DH.

Department of Health (2014) *One Chance to Get it Right*. London: DH.

Dimond, B. (2011) *Legal Aspects of Nursing and Healthcare*, 6th edn. Harlow: Pearson.

General Medical Council (2013) *Good Medical Practice*. London: GMC.

Health and Care Professions Council (2012) *Standards of Conduct, Performance and Ethics*. London: HCPC.

Khodyakov, D. and Carr, D. (2009) 'The impact of late-life parental death on adult sibling relationships: Do parents advance directives help or hurt?', *Research on Aging*, 31: 495–519.

Mason, J.K. and Laurie, G.T. (2011) *Mason and McCall Smith's Law and Medical Ethics*, 8th edn. Oxford: Oxford University Press.

Melia, K. (2014) *Ethics for Nursing and Healthcare Practice*. London: Sage.

National Council for Palliative Care (2007) *Artificial Nutrition and Hydration*. London: NCPC.

National Health Service (2011) *Capacity, Care Planning and Advance Care Planning in Life Limiting Illness: A Guide for Health and Social Care Staff*. London: DH.

Nursing and Midwifery Council (2015) *The Code: Professional Standards of Practice and Behaviour for Nurses and Midwives*. London: NMC.

Ogston-Tuck, S. (2014) 'Ethical issues in palliative and end of life care', in J. Nicol and B. Nyatanga (eds), *Palliative and End of Life Care in Nursing*. London: Sage, pp. 104–21.

Parliament (2005) *Mental Capacity Act 2005* Elizabeth II. London: The Stationary Office. Chapter 9. Available at: www.legislation.gov.uk/ukpga/2005/9/contents (accessed 15.7.2015).

Parliamentary and Health Service Ombudsman (2015) *Dying without Dignity: Investigations by the Parliamentary and Health Service Ombudsman into Complaints about End of Life Care*. London: Parliamentary and Health Service Ombudsman.

Stanley, K.J. and Zoloth-Dorfman, L. (2006) 'Ethical considerations', in B.R. Ferrell and N. Coyle (eds), *Textbook of Palliative Nursing*, 2nd edn. New York: Oxford University Press, pp. 1031–54.

Twycross, R. and Wilcock, A. (2001) *Symptom Management in Advanced Cancer*, 3rd edn. Oxford: Radcliffe Medical Press.

Watson, A.C. (2006) 'Urgent syndromes at the end of life', in B.R. Ferrell and N. Coyle (eds), *Textbook of Palliative Nursing*, 2nd edn. New York: Oxford University Press, pp. 443–66.

# 9
# End of life care

This chapter will explore:

- the philosophies underpinning end of life care
- issues which may present challenges in end of life care
- the legal and professional concepts which may support patient choice at the end of life
- the importance of understanding the 'individual,' recognising and establishing their specific needs.

## What is end of life care planning?

There is little doubt that end of life care is important to everyone. People generally recognise that both they themselves and those around them may have specific fears, wishes or requests when it comes to end of life care. Starting any discussion surrounding end of life care can incite anxiety amongst health and social care professionals for a number of reasons, which may include the consideration of one's own mortality (Cialkowska-Rysz and Dzierzanowski 2013; Brown et al. 2009). As we are faced with an increasingly aging population (NAO 2008), the demand for high-quality end of life care for those with life-limiting illness, including cancer, may be amplified. This does not negate the need to maintain or even improve the end of life care provision that a patient should expect and have a right to. They should receive the highest quality care no matter what diagnosis, geographical area, age or socioeconomic status; in addition, marginalised groups (e.g. travellers, prison population) should have equal access to end of life care (National Council for Palliative Care 2014). Quality requirement 9 in the *National Service Framework for Long Term Conditions* (DH 2005) states that holistic end of life care is paramount for people living with a long-term condition (LTC). This standard is reiterated throughout the UK (NHS Scotland 2009; Welsh Government 2014; Long Term Conditions Alliance Northern Ireland 2008).

# When to initiate end of life care planning

Deciding when to initiate palliative and end of life care is a shared anxiety for the healthcare team. The Gold Standards Framework (2006) *Prognostic Indicator Guidance* provides direction through the form of questioning (see Figure 9.1), and acts as a prompt to start discussing end of life care wishes if the team feels that the patient's health is deteriorating. For example, the guidance suggests you start with the 'surprise' question:

- Would you be surprised if this person died within the next 6–12 months?

If the answer is no, then discussions surrounding wishes at the end of life should be initiated, including choices surrounding place of care and preferred place of death.

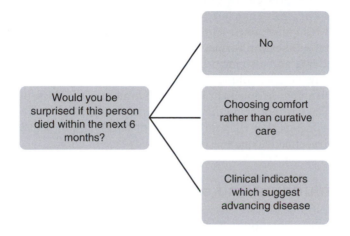

**Figure 9.1**    Prognostic indicator guidance (Gold Standards Framework 2006)

A second prompt would be if the individual with advancing disease chooses comfort rather than curative care. The third point of guidance concerns clinical indicators: those which would indicate advancing disease or deteriorating condition, such as increasing tumour markers in a patient with cancer (these are markers measured through blood testing and a rise often occurs in response to advancing and progressing cancer. There are specific markers for specific cancers, e.g. prostate specific antigen for prostate cancer). The indicators identified in the guidance are to help ascertain those who are nearing the end of life to ensure that they receive the support, care and interventions which may aid a 'good death', rather than patients experiencing urgent care that has not been anticipated and hence the patient has very little time to think about what they would want, or worse still no time to discuss their wishes. Other indicators include: general physical decline, which may be due to disease burden; decreasing response to treatment, indicating advancing disease escaping control of available treatments; and progressive weight loss, which may be due to increasing fatigue through advancing disease, or in some cases where cancer causes a rise in metabolic rate. Within the prognostic indicator guidance

(Gold Standards Framework 2006) there are 11 general indicators as well as other disease-specific indicators (e.g. heart disease, cancer, Parkinson's disease etc.), which should increase the validity and reliability of the guidance. Its purpose is to support decisions which are often difficult to discuss and to present emotive situations requiring effective, sensitive communication skills.

With the increasing demands for complex end of life care, any provision may require well-coordinated interprofessional end of life care. This may be delivered in a number of settings ranging from care at home to a variety of private and voluntary organisations (e.g. hospices, nursing homes, a patient's own home, acute or rehabilitation hospital settings). Care is not only provided by health and social care professionals but also by informal carers who may have their own specific needs too (see Chapter 5). The National Audit Office (2008) identified a number of barriers to high-quality end of life care, including lack of recognition that a person was approaching end of life, which may be addressed with the Gold Standards Framework (2006) guidance (Thomas 2003). The draft guideline from NICE (2015) has recommendations which include how to recognise when someone is approaching the end of life, so when released in its full publication format it may help health and social care staff to provide appropriate care and also identify when end of life discussions may be required. Other reasons may include: failure to communicate effectively to carers/family; a lack of end of care planning; people kept in hospital unnecessarily; lack of education and knowledge; and lack of understanding surrounding commissioning resources for end of life care. This means that there are significant challenges in delivering end of life care in a proactive, effective manner in a patient's place of choice.

## Issues surrounding end of life care planning

Guidance and policies relating to end of life care have been and continue to be introduced in an attempt to guide staff and ensure access to high-level palliative and end of life care (DH 2008; NAO 2008; DH 2014a; NICE 2015). The General Medical Council stated that individuals encounter barriers to high-quality end of life care for a number of reasons, which may include lack of awareness regarding available support but also may be due to physical or communication problems (2010). Despite this, ethical principles and legislation underpins not only medical practitioners, but also nurses: see the Nursing and Midwifery Council's *The Code* (2015), the Health Care and Professions Council *Council Standards for Performance and Ethics* (2008) and the General Pharmaceutical Council's *Standards of Conduct, Ethics and Performance* (2012). They all state that respect for the individual, maintaining their dignity and providing fair treatment to all requiring care is obligatory policy and guidance concurred with the use of a pathway for end of life care referred to as the Liverpool Care Pathway (Independent Review 2013) (DH 2008; NAO 2008; NICE 2004).

The recommendations from the published *More Care, Less Pathway* (Independent Review 2013) identified five key priorities to ensure that caring for the patient is focused on their specific needs and with the carer(s) and relatives included where possible so that they can be supported though the journey:

1. This possibility is recognised and communicated clearly, decisions made and actions taken in accordance with the person's needs and wishes, and these are regularly reviewed and decisions revised accordingly.
2. Sensitive communication takes place between staff and the dying person, and those identified as important to them.
3. The dying person, and those identified as important to them, are involved in decisions about treatment and care to the extent that the dying person wants.
4. The needs of families and others identified as important to the dying person are actively explored, respected and met as far as possible.
5. An individual plan of care, which includes food and drink, symptom control and psychological, social and spiritual support, is agreed, co-ordinated and delivered with compassion. (DH 2014a: 7)

# Why is end of life care planning important?

> This possibility is recognised and communicated clearly, decisions made and actions taken in accordance with the person's needs and wishes, and these are regularly reviewed and decisions revised accordingly. (DH 2014a: 7)

High-quality end of life care will be a challenge and costly. Decisions need to be made regarding whether it is worth the investment (Seymour and Horne 2013). The decision may already be made as the general public are demanding that level of care for their loved ones (Parliamentary and Health Service Ombudsmen 2015). To suggest that it may not be worth investing in is likely to be an unpopular decision, especially as the need for this level of care is likely to rise. What we may have to do is work in a much more collaborative way, foster support to our colleagues and provide formal and informal education at every available opportunity. Seeking those educational opportunities and reflecting on our practice is the responsibility of every healthcare professional (NICE 2015; NMC 2015).

---

### 👥 Case scenario: Rita

Rita, aged 55, had advanced breast cancer. Her district nurse and GP felt her prognosis was poor and that she was reaching the end of life, therefore they decided to have an open and honest discussion with Rita. She felt supported and was encouraged to make decisions about her end of life care wishes. The Macmillan nurse had also become involved in Rita's care due to complex symptom issues. Rita discussed her wishes with her husband and the district nurse. She stated that she did not want to be in pain or distressed as she approached the end of life so would want effective symptom

*(Continued)*

*(Continued)*

management measures (e.g. sedation) if necessary. She did not want to die at home but wanted the security of the hospice as she had spent some time there having her symptoms treated, and she wanted her husband to remain with her. She discussed her funeral and that she wanted her husband Derek to go on and live life to the full for her. Rita died in the hospice with her husband laid next to her, pain free and peaceful.

## Reflection points

- How did Rita exercise autonomy?
- How did you feel about Rita's death?
- How would you feel if you had been involved in Rita's care?
- What do you think of Derek's experience?
- What care management and delivery facilitated Rita to die as she did?

Patients have the right to self-determination: in other words, their autonomy should be maximised. When approaching the end of life, a patient's right to make decisions rather than decisions being made for them is even more crucial to facilitate a patient-centred experience. Care delivered in conflict with the patient's wishes falls far short of what they deserve, therefore clear communication surrounding their disease and likely care needs is paramount to limit stress and anxiety (Skilbeck and Payne 2003). Rita was able to be explicit about her needs and wishes for both herself and her husband. This should have a very positive effect on Derek's bereavement experience, and also on the nurses and other health and social care professionals who were involved in making Rita's decisions and needs happen. The care plan should also be updated regularly to ensure that the patient has not changed their mind and that the care meets their needs (see Chapter 4 for further discussion surrounding care planning).

## The patient

Research has been undertaken to determine individual patient's views surrounding end of life care (Horne et al. 2012; Office of National Statistics 2013; Gomes et al. 2011). There are commonalities (e.g. be pain free, dying in the place of their choice, wanting to concentrate on living rather than dying), but one may be presented with very specific requests which are unique to the individual (e.g. having their ashes sprinkled in a specific place, the desire to experience a small amount of pain so that they know they are still alive). Care such as this should be non-judgemental even if it appears unorthodox or at odds with one's own perceptions.

*Actions for End of Life Care* (NHS 2014) is a strategy which hopes to deliver targets and guidance to enable those reaching the end of life to have a high-quality end of life care experience. This guidance was born out of engagement with patients, carers, families, volunteers, health and social care professionals and those with a high interest in end of life care which includes organisations responsible for delivering this care. The guidance purports that 75 per cent of deaths are expected, therefore with adequate education and time to provide care and support then the experience at the end of life should be of a high standard and be responsive to the specific needs of the individual, no matter whether it is provided by specialist or non-specialist services. Unmet need has been identified in approximately 170,000 people resulting in referral to specialist palliative care teams, with an increasing need identified in those with non-cancer conditions and harder to reach populations.

 ## Case scenario: Ethel

Ethel, aged 80, has heart failure. She is breathless with bilateral leg oedema and fears that things are getting worse. She is anxious and frightened about the future and feels life is difficult as she cannot do the things she enjoys doing. She is anxious about leaving the house and is getting quite low in mood. She feels fatigued and has experienced some chest pain. She sees her GP for her regular medication reviews but other than that she has no contact with professionals.

## Reflection points

Ethel is clearly deteriorating, so consider:

- What unmet needs do you think Ethel has?
- How could you support Ethel?
- How could you empower Ethel?

Unmet needs can be obvious (e.g. a patient with unresolved cancer pain or having difficulty coming to terms with treatment failure for lung cancer), but, in contrast, unmet needs may be less clear for those with non-cancer conditions, perhaps due to the fact that prognosis is difficult to predict. With Ethel's fear, anxiety, fatigue and inability to function, as well as her physical symptoms, it is clear that she has significant unmet needs. By 2025 the number living with LTCs is expected to rise to 18 million (NHS 2014), and increasing complexity arises when a patient may have two or more LTCs, making management of their deteriorating conditions a challenge and the potential for unmet need a greater problem.

## Case scenario: Hetty

Hetty, aged 55, has a diagnosis of motor neurone disease, she is deteriorating slowly but her ability to swallow is becoming affected. The consultant discusses artificial nutrition with Hetty. She declines and says she would rather let nature take its course than prolong her suffering. The consultant feels this is the wrong decision and tries to persuade Hetty to go ahead with the insertion of a percutaneous endoscopic gastrostomy feeding tube (PEG) to allow artificial nutrition to be delivered. His reason is that Hetty's disease appears to be reasonably slow in comparison with many other patients he has come across, so feels that this will have a significant affect on Hetty's life expectancy. Hetty reiterates her decision and refuses treatment.

## Reflection points

- Can you see Hetty's point of view?
- How can you be sure Hetty is doing it for the right reason?
- What would be the right reason?
- What do you think of the consultant's approach?

Hetty may feel emotionally, psychologically, spiritually and physically exhausted as having a life-limiting illness may induce overwhelming fatigue and stress, not only on the patient but on the relatives and carers too (see Chapter 5 for carer burden). One needs to ensure that Hetty is making the decision because she feels her quality of life is such that the future holds no hope and her suffering is too much to bear despite effective symptom management. If it was to reduce carer burden or because she feels she's being a trouble, then one may argue that this would not be the 'right reason'. Taking time to find out the reasons for a patient's choices are paramount in trying to determine their motivation and reasoning behind decisions made, just as it is important to determine their worries and anxieties. Trying to acknowledge and identify reversible symptoms and maintain some hope can make a significant difference to a patient's quality of life.

> The dying person, and those identified as important to them, are involved in decisions about treatment and care to the extent that the dying person wants. (DH 2014b: 7)

Giving people a chance to say what they want is vital as time may be limited and cannot be recaptured at a later date. As nurses we are bound by the NMC principles and standards (NMC 2015) to ensure that patients are empowered, and this is done through the provision of information which has been delivered effectively and in an understandable manner using appropriate resources if required, supporting the patient and encouraging them to make decisions about type of treatment or place of treatment as long as it is practicable. Difficulties come when a patient's cognitive function deteriorates and it becomes increasingly difficult to gain consent or determine their wishes for future care.

---

### 👥 Case scenario: Gerald

Gerald, aged 52, was admitted to the nursing home for end of life care. He had no relatives, no lasting power of attorney or advanced decision to refuse treatment. Unfortunately Gerald had advanced dementia and he was deemed to lack capacity. The staff tried to find out more about Gerald so that they could tailor Gerald's end of life care around his wishes and preferences. They contacted his GP who had very little information about Gerald other than about his period of illness. His friend who visited could offer little of what Gerald would have wanted as their chats revolved around football and work until he deteriorated. However, his friend carried on visiting even when the chats ceased.

---

## Reflection points

- Gerald did not have an advanced decision to refuse treatment; what effect will this have on his care?
- How can this affect the nurses' role?
- What do you think the nurses should do in this situation?
- What about a 'do not attempt resuscitation' order?

---

End of life care involves delivering high-quality care to those who are in the last few days or weeks of life. The fact that there were no explicit wishes from Gerald does not mean that the healthcare team cannot work in his best interest (see Chapter 8 for further discussion). Thinking about whether it would be appropriate to attempt to resuscitate Gerald if he sustained a cardiac arrest is one of the clinical decisions that can insight great stress. Robinson et al. (2007) found in their study that nurses experienced greater stress surrounding these decisions than their medical colleagues, and this may be due, in part, to a lack of confidence in discussing it (Sulmasy et al. 2008), uncertainties about family involvement, and at times lack of a trusting relationship with the doctor involved in the decision-making process (Silén et al. 2008; Thacker 2008). Undoubtedly having an honest discussion with the patient and/or their carer/relatives can help ensure that the right decision is made for that particular individual, as what should be considered is not only whether it has a chance of being successful (i.e. the patient surviving the arrest) but also the quality of life preceding the event and likely quality of life post-resuscitation.

Ensuring that Gerald is pain free and not suffering is paramount. Encouraging his friend to bring items from Gerald's home if that hasn't already been done may make Gerald feel more comfortable and the environment less alien to him. In an ideal world, a professional should have helped Gerald record his wishes for end of life care at an appropriate point, but identifying that point is a difficult task and perhaps a principle reason why so many patients with a non-cancer diagnosis have not had the opportunity to discuss end of life and plan the care alongside a healthcare professional.

## The legal concepts

Ensuring that people have the opportunity to relay their wishes regarding end of life treatment and care can be facilitated in a more formal manner. 'Advanced directives' are an advanced decision to refuse treatment (Parliament 2005: s24). A patient cannot demand treatment. The decision has to be specific in order to reduce any uncertainty for those charged with caring for someone when they are unable to voice their wishes or consent to treatment (see Chapter 8 for a more comprehensive discussion surrounding the legal and ethical issues at the end of life).

---

### 👥 Case scenario: Edna

Edna, aged 72, was diagnosed with chronic obstructive pulmonary disease and had suffered a number of exacerbations. She had been seen in clinic by her physician and he suggested that she have a think about what she would like if she became very unwell. Edna went home and drafted a letter and stated that this was her advance decision to refuse treatment. Her specific wishes included no ventilating in the event of her deterioration. She placed her advance decision in a safe place at home. Several weeks later she became extremely breathless, she felt frightened and knew this was much worse than before. She dialled 999 and got out her advance decision to refuse treatment for the ambulance crew. Shortly after they arrived, Edna deteriorated, she was unrousable and her oxygen saturation was extremely low, indicating a life-threatening event.

The ambulance crew looked at the advance decision to refuse treatment. Edna was deteriorating and she needed ventilating. The letter itself had not been witnessed. One of the ethical and legal challenges faced by the paramedics was that the letter did not specify the type of ventilation she was refusing either, they did not know Edna personally, and therefore working in her best interest and with some doubt regarding whether she meant invasive ventilation rather than non-invasive ventilation and the validity of the decision, they proceeded to prepare for non-invasive ventilation and get Edna to hospital as quickly as possible together with her advance decision to refuse treatment.

**Reflection points**

- What more could the physician have done to help Edna?
- Do you think the ambulance staff made the right decision?
- Consider the ethical implications of applying non-invasive ventilation.

The physician, whilst he started the discussion with Edna about end of life care wishes, provided very little information surrounding how she could ensure that her wishes were carried out. The advance decision to refuse treatment should be clear regarding wishes at the end of life (Brown and Vaughan 2013) and without ambiguity. Unfortunately 'no ventilation' may not be specific enough for staff to withhold treatment, as it would almost certainly result in the demise of the patient. In this situation the staff acted correctly, but once Edna recovered she would need to be given some help and support regarding her advance decision to refuse treatment. To be valid the decision should be witnessed and must also state 'even if my life is at risk' (Department of Constitutional Affairs 2007), which it wasn't in Edna's case.

The difficulties with end of life care lie with the fact that death may be imminent and withdrawal or withholding treatment may result in premature deterioration, but in some circumstances to treat may cause more pain and distress than to not treat. Article 8 of the Human Rights Act 1998, 'respect for private and family life', gives individuals the right for moral autonomy. The Mental Capacity Act (Parliament 2005) has provided further support to individuals in order that they maintain their autonomy. Its premise is that one should assume capacity and take every possible opportunity to allow a patient to make decisions. If a patient has a condition whereby their capacity is expected to diminish (e.g. Alzheimer's disease), then having discussions about their wishes and the use of advance decisions to refuse treatment can help to ensure a patient's expressed wishes are acknowledged, planned for and achieved where possible (see Chapter 8 for further discussion about legal and ethical issues at the end of life).

## Communication at the end of life

Sensitive communication takes place between staff and the dying person, and those identified as important to them. (DH 2014b: 7)

As discussed in Chapter 7, communication when a person has reached the palliative phase of illness can incur difficult conversations and may require advanced skills and understanding surrounding the patient's specific needs and concerns. Discussing end of life care requires constant reiteration, checking and information provision to ensure that there is a mutual understanding and awareness regarding the current issues in the patient's journey, the plan of care, and any new symptoms or concerns that may present. Dahlin and Giansiracusa (2006) suggest that communication in palliative care sets the tone for all the care which may be required because without effective communication, patients and relatives may be left feeling isolated, unaware of the current situation presented and lacking trust in those providing care.

A study examining carer's and relative's experience of care identified some common issues. These revolved around not being told that that their loved ones were dying, which caused great distress and in some cases complicated their grief (NHS 2014). As a result guidance was developed which includes a request that doctors must discuss prognosis with the patient where possible and potentially their loved ones as soon as it becomes clear that the patient may die relatively soon. In addition to communicating this news, the healthcare team should ensure that the patient is as comfortable as possible, with distressing symptoms assessed and discussed, with any reversible causes treated and irreversible causes palliated. 'Treatment' means to reverse the cause; for example, hypercalcaemia can present in people nearing end of life but may be distressing in its initial stages with the onset of confusion and so on. Reversing the hypercalcaemia with medication can reduce the calcium, thereby treating the cause resulting in symptom relief. Delirium at the end of life could occur for a number of reasons (e.g. infection, medication, other pathologies), but if a patient is very close to end of life it may be unethical to try to investigate as they may die before a cause is determined, causing the patient unnecessary suffering. Treating the delirium via palliative measures would be to treat the symptom rather than the cause. It is a case of 'what is the most appropriate treatment?' (Twycross and Wilcock 2001: 4).

To ascertain any troublesome or distressing symptoms or suffering, effective communication is needed to elicit this information and attempt to resolve it through discussion with the patient (Buckman 2001). In addition, effective listening skills are important so that one can try to understand the contributing factors and address the patient's concerns, as these may be quite complex and more than a simple set of symptoms to treat.

> The needs of families and others identified as important to the dying person are actively explored, respected and met as far as possible. (DH 2014b: 7)

Suffering is not limited to those at the end of life, it is distressing for loved ones and carers too. Carers may have already endured a distressing time in caring for their loved one, and this could have been for a protracted period of time. Many carers have significant physical, psychological, spiritual and social consequences to caring (HM Government 2008; Gaugler et al. 2005; Nijboer et al. 1998; Stroebe et al. 2007; Barrow and Harrison 2005) (see Chapter 5). Ensuring that they do not feel uninvolved or marginalised when prioritising care for the patient should be considered, especially if they have coped alone for some time. Feeling rejected and uninvolved may lead to feelings of inadequacy as professionals 'take over'. This could have negative effects on their bereavement journey.

# Symptom management at the end of life

Distressing symptoms at the end of life can be diverse and they may result in not only physical effects but also psychological, spiritual and social consequences. If effective symptom management is achieved at the end of life, perceptions of care may be more positive than if a loved one was seen to be suffering and in some distress (NICE 2012). Pain control is synonymous with palliative and end of life care and pain is the symptom that elicits a great deal of fear (Caraceni and Weinstein 2001). Assessing pain requires a robust approach whereby the type and cause of pain should be elicited where possible in order to attempt to provide appropriate interventions. These interventions may be pharmacological or non-pharmacological. The non-pharmacological intervention may comprise acupuncture, reflexology, psychologist input for example, but other treatments could include radiotherapy, chemotherapy or surgical interventions in an attempt to treat distressing pain.

> An individual plan of care, which includes food and drink, symptom control and psychological, social and spiritual support, is agreed, co-ordinated and delivered with compassion.
> (DH 2014b: 7)

Assessment tools can help to ensure that a comprehensive approach is adopted. One tool that may be helpful to aid the assessment for patients with palliative care needs is the PEPSI COLA aide memoire (Gold Standards Framework Programme 2014; Thomas 2003). This incorporates the full holistic assessment and acknowledges the unique needs of a patient and that symptoms are very unlikely to be of a physical nature alone (see Figure 9.2).

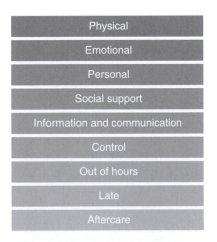

**Figure 9.2** The PEPSI COLA domains (Thomas 2003)

PEPSI COLA is the holistic assessment tool recommended as part of the GSF programme in Primary Care, care homes, hospitals and others developed by Professor Keri Thomas and team. For details, please visit www.goldstandardsframework.co.uk or email info@gsfcentre.co.uk.

These prompts lead the healthcare professional through the full holistic assessment, but one needs to be familiar with what may need discussing; for example, in the emotional domain one should be discussing the psychological wellbeing of the individual, and cue questions such as 'What is worrying you the most?' may be helpful in order to get some discussion started (Pettifer 2013). Education and training may be required prior to adopting such tools in practice to ensure that they are used appropriately and to their full potential in aiding a comprehensive approach (see Chapter 3 for further discussion surrounding holistic assessment).

It is the extent of the problems or symptoms which make end of life care a challenge, and it is this complexity that may necessitate the involvement of the specialist palliative care team. Increasing the skills and knowledge of health and social care staff should be a priority as the increasing incidence of those suffering with more than one LTC may exacerbate such complex symptom presentations. Ensuring that the healthcare professional performing the assessment has the skills to identify issues and symptoms but also to make sense of what is happening may induce confidence from those being cared for.

A compassionate and non-judgmental approach is crucial in allowing the patient to be open and honest. This engagement may be the only opportunity to record a patient's concerns and take a history resulting in a comprehensive understanding of the care needs because patients may deteriorate rapidly. A poor or less than adequate assessment may leave those being cared for feeling anxious, upset or frustrated that they are misunderstood or not listened to. The healthcare professional may feel inadequate or guilty if they know that their assessment did not meet the patient's needs. Empowering the patient and maintaining their autonomy whilst being realistic about what may be achieved will help generate the therapeutic relationship that fosters a supportive role and may make a patient's experience at the end of life a fulfilled one where wishes are respected and dignity is maintained.

## Pain

There are several distressing symptoms which may require intervention as one approaches end of life (e.g. fatigue, anorexia, nausea, constipation and depression). Using a comprehensive assessment tool as identified earlier can help in the development of a treatment or intervention strategy and for planning care. Some symptoms can present significant challenges to the health and social care professional (e.g. complex pain presentations). Pain may be synonymous with death and dying in those with a cancer or non-cancer related life-limiting condition as they approach end of life. The World Health Organization (2004) introduced the analgesic ladder and guidance surrounding pain relief for those suffering with chronic pain. It suggests that the effective way to deliver pain relief is 'by the mouth, by the clock, by the individual, by the analgesic ladder' (WHO 2004). 'By the mouth' means that wherever possible, analgesia should be delivered orally but when this is no longer feasible, then the most appropriate and least invasive route of administration should be adopted. The 'ladder' refers to the administration of non-opioids (e.g. paracetamol) initially, moving up to mild opioids (e.g. codeine) if still unresolved, then to strong opioids (e.g. morphine). 'By the clock' means that analgesia should be delivered on a regular basis if the patient is reporting recurrent pain rather than administering on an ad hoc basis. Analgesia should be administered after a comprehensive assessment taking a history and using diagnostic reasoning in order to ascertain probable cause and route of pain, establishing provocative (what makes it worse?) and palliative (what makes it better?) factors. To maximise effect a non-opioid may be given alongside a mild opioid (e.g. codeine and paracetamol) (WHO 2004). Some pain can be very complex, with a mixture of presentations (e.g. muscular pain but with accompanying sharp or shooting pain) that may require different approaches for the different pains. The use of anti-inflammatory agents may be useful alongside a non-opioid, mild opioid or strong opioid for bone pain, for example (Twycross and Wilcock 2001).

 ## Case scenario: Hector

Hector, aged 52, presented to the outpatient clinic with a history of weight loss and back pain. He underwent a bone scan and returned for the result. The doctor relays some bad news and informs Hector that he has bone metastases but they are unsure where the primary cancer is situated. The main concern currently is his pain. This is causing him severe distress and inducing significant disruption to his life. He cannot sleep and has been unable to work, which has caused great anxiety as he is self-employed and so has no income. His quality of life has diminished in all aspects as a result of his pain and subsequent diagnosis. He is devastated and his concern is for his wife and children. They refer him to the specialist palliative care team for assessment.

## Reflection points

- What tools could you utilise in order to assess Hector?
- What are the priorities and how are you going to determine what they are?
- What other professional teams could you involve to help Hector?

Hector has a number of issues which cannot be separated into physical, psychological, spiritual and social. His symptoms and anxieties are having an effect on him as a whole. A holistic assessment is vital, and these situations and presentations where a patient is extremely distressed for a number of reasons reinforce the importance of holistic assessment and care planning (see Chapters 3 and 4). Determining Hector's priorities and getting him to make decisions about treatment should be core to effective, individualised care planning. Deciding which symptom should take precedence is Hector's decision, not that of the healthcare professional.

Pain is just one symptom that may present itself as a patient reaches the end of life and, as already identified, symptoms are not only of a physical nature but may also be multidimensional and have significant effects on a patient's overall quality of life. It is important, therefore, that one takes time to gain a full history and identify and discuss the impact these symptoms are having on their life, using a tool like the PEPSI COLA aide memoire (Gold Standards Framework Programme 2014; Thomas 2003).

## Conclusion

Being involved in end of life care is a privilege and the importance that high-quality delivery can have on the patient and their loved ones cannot be underestimated. We, as health and social care professionals, have the opportunity to make a real difference. Similar to the guidance surrounding *Making Every Contact Count* (DH 2014a), which focuses on health promotion and the opportunity to discuss general health needs, *Every Moment Counts* addresses the need for person-centred care and was produced in collaboration with National Voices (National Council for Palliative Care 2015). Making every moment count with a patient at the end of life is crucial as this may be the last contact a health or social care professional has with the dying patient, making it the last thing that anyone does for them. Ensuring that care remains patient-centred and maximising any opportunity to hear the patient's wishes and preferences is fundamental when a patient approaches the end of their life.

## Recommended reading

Brown, M. and Vaughan, C. (2013) 'Care at the end of life: How policy and the law support practice', *British Journal of Nursing*, 22: 10.

Buckman, R. (2001) 'Communication skills in palliative care', *Neurology Clinician*, 19: 989–1004.

Department of Health (2014) *One Chance to Get it Right: How Health and Care Organisations Should Care for People in the Last Days of their Life*. London: DH.

Gold Standards Framework Programme (2006) *Prognostic Indicator Guidance to Aid Identification of Adult Patients with Advanced Disease in the Last Months/Year of Life, Who are in Need of Supportive and Palliative Care*, Version 1.24 Prognostic Indicator Paper vs 1.21. Birmingham: Gold Standards Framework. Available at: www. goldstandardsframework.org.uk (accessed 11.6.15).

## References

Barrow, S. and Harrison, R.A. (2005) 'Unsung heroes who put their lives at risk? Informal caring, health and neighbourhood attachment', *Journal of Public Health*, 27(3): 292–7.

Brown, M. and Vaughan, C. (2013) 'Care at the end of life: How policy and the law support practice', *British Journal of Nursing*, 22: 10.

Brown, R., Dunn, S., Byrnes, K., Morris, R., Heinrich, P. and Shaw, J. (2009) 'Doctors' stress responses and poor communication performance in simulated bad-news consultations, *Academic Medicine*, 84(11): 1595–602.

Buckman, R. (2001) 'Communication skills in palliative care', *Neurology Clinician*, 19: 989–1004.

Caraceni, A. and Weinstein, S.M. (2001) 'Classification of cancer pain syndromes', *Oncology*, 15(12): 1627–40.

Cialkowska-Rysz, A. and Dzierzanowski, T. (2013) 'Personal fear of death affects the proper process of breaking bad news', *Archives of Medical Science*, 9(1): 127–31.

Dahlin, C.M. and Giansiracusa, D.F. (2006) 'Communication in palliative care', in B. R. Ferrell and N. Coyle (eds), *Textbook of Palliative Nursing*. New York: Oxford University Press, pp. 67–94.

Department for Constitutional Affairs (2007) *Mental Capacity Act 2005: Code of Practice*. London: The Stationery Office.

Department of Health (2005) *The National Service Framework for Long Term Conditions*. London: DH.

Department of Health (2008) *End of Life Care Strategy*. London: DH.

Department of Health (2014a) *Making Every Contact Count*. London: DH.

Department of Health (2014b) *One Chance to Get it Right: How Health and Care Organisations Should Care for People in the Last Days of their Life*. London: DH.

Gaugler, J.E., Hanna, N., Linder, J., Given, C.W., Tolber, V., Katernia, R. and Regine, W.F. (2005) 'Cancer care giving and subjective stress: a multi-site, multi-dimensional analysis', *Psycho-Oncology*, 14(9): 771–85.

General Medical Council (2010) *Treatment Towards the End of Life: Good Practice in Decision Making*. Manchester: General Medical Council.

General Pharmaceutical Council (2012) *Standards of Conduct, Ethics and Performance*. London: GPC.

Gold Standards Framework Programme (2006) *Prognostic Indicator Guidance to Aid Identification of Adult Patients with Advanced Disease in the Last Months/Year of Life, Who are in Need of Supportive and Palliative Care*, Version 1.24 Prognostic Indicator Paper vs 1.21. Birmingham: Gold Standards Framework. Available at: www.goldstandardsframework.org. uk (accessed 11.6.15).

Gold Standards Framework Programme (2014) *Holistic Checklist: PEPSI COLA Aide Memoire*. Birmingham: Gold Standards Framework. Available at: www.goldstandards framework.org.uk/cd-content/uploads/files/Library%2C%20Tools%20%26%20 resources/SCR4%20Pepsi%20cola.pdf (accessed 11.6.15).

Gomes, B., Calanzani, N. and Higginson, I.J. (2011) *Local Preferences and Place of Death in Regions within England 2010*. London: Cecily Saunders Foundation.

Health Care and Professions Council (2008) *Council Standards for Performance and Ethics*. London: HCPC.

HM Government (2008) *Carers at the Heart of the 21st Century: Families and Communities*. London: DH.

Horne, G., Seymour, J. and Payne, S. (2012) 'Maintaining integrity in the face of death: A grounded theory to explain the perspectives of people affected by lung cancer about the expression of wishes for end of life care', *International Journal of Nursing Studies*, 49: 718–26.

Human Rights Act (1998) *Chapter 42*. London: The Stationery Office.

Independent Review of the Liverpool Care Pathway Panel (2013) *More Care, Less Pathway: A Review of the Liverpool Care Pathway*. London: DH.

Long Term Conditions Alliance Northern Ireland (2008) *Responses to Proposals for Health and Social Care Reform in Northern Ireland*. Available at: www.ltcani.org.uk/resources/ Response-NHS-reforms-May08.pdf (accessed 8.12.14).

National Audit Office (2008) *End of Life Care*. London: The Stationery Office.

National Council for Palliative Care (2014) *About NCPC*. London: NCPC. Available at: www.ncpc.org.uk/ (accessed 3.1.14).

National Council for Palliative Care (2015) *Every Moment Counts: A Narrative for Person-centred Coordinated Care for People Near the End of Life*. London: National Voices.

National Health Service (2014) *Actions for End of Life Care: 2014–16*. London: DH.

National Health Service Scotland (2009) *Long Term Conditions Collaborative: High Impact Changes*. Edinburgh: NHSS.

National Institute for Health and Care Excellence (2004) *Guidance on Cancer Services Improving Supportive and Palliative Care for Adults with Cancer: The Manual*. London: NICE.

National Institute for Health and Care Excellence (2012) *Opioids in Palliative Care: Safe and Effective Prescribing of Strong Opioids for Pain in Palliative Care of Adults*. London: NICE.

National Institute for Health and Care Excellence (2015) *Care of the Dying Adult: Guidance in Progress*. London: NICE. Available at: www.nice.org.uk/guidance/indevelopment/gid-cgwave0694 (accessed 20 August 2015).

Nijboer, C., Templaar, R., Sanderman, R., Triemstra, M., Spruijt, R.J. and Van Den Bos, G.A. (1998) 'Cancer and care giving: The impact on the caregiver's health', *Psycho-Oncology*, 7: 3–13.

Nursing and Midwifery Council (2015) *The Code: Professional Standards of Practice and Behaviour for Nurses and Midwives*. London: NMC.

Office for National Statistics (2013) *National Survey of Bereaved People (VOICES-SF)*, 2013. London: ONS. Available at: www.ons.gov.uk/ons/rel/subnational-health1/national-survey-of-bereaved-people--voices-/2013/stb---national-survey-of-bereaved-people--voices-.html (accessed 5.1.15).

Parliament (2005) *Mental Capacity Act 2005 Elizabeth II*. London: The Stationary Office. Chapter 9. Available at: www.legislation.gov.uk/ukpga/2005/9/contents (accessed 11.6.15).

Parliamentary and Health Service Ombudsman (2015) *Dying without Dignity: Investigations by the Parliamentary and Health Service Ombudsman into Complaints about End of Life Care*. London: Parliamentary and Health Service Ombudsman.

Pettifer, A. (2013) 'Assessing holistic needs', in J. De Souza and A. Pettifer (eds), *End of Life Nursing Care: A Guide for Best Practice*. London: Sage, pp. 16–34.

Robinson, F., Cupples, M. and Corrigan, M. (2007) 'Implementing a resuscitation policy for patients at the end of life in an acute hospital setting: Qualitative study', *Palliative Medicine*, 21: 305–12.

Silén, M., Svantesson, M. and Ahlstrom, G. (2008) 'Nurses' conceptions of decision making concerning life-sustaining treatment', *Nursing Ethics*, 15: 160–73.

Skilbeck, J. and Payne, S. (2003) 'Emotional support and the role of the clinical nurse specialist in palliative care', *Journal of Advanced Nursing*, 43(5): 521–30.

Stroebe, M., Schut, H. and Stroebe, W. (2007) 'Health outcomes of bereavement', *Lancet*, 370: 1960–73.

Sulmasy, D.P., He, M.K., McAuley, R. and Ury, W.A. (2008) 'Beliefs and attitudes of nurses and physicians about do not resuscitate orders and who should speak to patients and families about them', *Critical Care Medicine*, 36: 1817–22.

Thacker, K.S. (2008) 'Nurses' advocacy behaviors in end-of-life nursing care', *Nursing Ethics*, 15: 174–85.

Thomas, K. (2003) *Caring for the Dying at Home: Companions on the Journey*. Oxford: Radcliffe Medical Press.

Twycross, R. and Wilcock, A. (2001) *Symptom Management in Advanced Cancer*, 3rd edn. Oxford: Radcliffe Medical Press.

Welsh Government (2014) *End of Life Care Delivery Plan*. Cardiff: Welsh Government. Available at: http://gov.wales/topics/health/nhswales/plans/end-of-life-care/?lang=en (accessed 11.6.15).

World Health Organization (2004) *Palliative Care and Symptom Management and End of Life Care: Integrated Management of Adolescent and Adult Illness*. Geneva: WHO.

# 10

# Death and dying

This chapter will explore:

- the predictability of death
- assessment and its importance in caring for those at the end of life
- signs and symptoms which may indicate that death is approaching
- what constitutes a good death
- pain management in the last days or weeks of life
- dignity in death
- grief and grief models.

How people die remains in the memory of those that live on. (Saunders 1976)

## Background

Individuals have a right to be informed about their prognosis (Cialkowska-Rysz and Dzierzanowski 2013; NICE 2011). It gives them the opportunity not only to deal with their affairs but also to say goodbye to loved ones. Undoubtedly we would all desire a 'good death' for ourselves and, from a professional stance, this is what we would like to achieve when caring for our patients as they approach the end of life (Miyashita et al. 2015; Cagle et al. 2015; Cipolletta and Oprandi 2014). Trying to establish what that should consist of continues to challenge researchers and theorists (Baldwin and Woodhouse 2011; Steinhauser et al. 2000), but it is likely to be different for each and every one of us and may in fact change over time or when faced with distressing diagnoses or disease. The Parliamentary and Health Service Ombudsman (2015) has identified a number of issues that require urgent attention so that suffering at the end of life no longer happens (e.g. lack of recognition that someone is dying).

Age Concern (1999) identified that in order to achieve a good death, being aware of its imminence was imperative so that one could make plans, but being free from pain and other distressing symptoms also appear to be a consistent theme within the literature (Baldwin and Woodhouse 2011). Although culture may play some part in determining what constitutes a 'good death,' Cipolletta and Oprandi (2014) investigated experiences amongst a variety of healthcare professionals surrounding end of life care in Italy. They identified that, culturally, the sanctity of life was far more important than a patient's quality of life, and they reported that many patients who are nursed in hospital at the end of life suffer due to the inadequacies in the care delivered and therefore a 'good death' was not achieved in some cases. Deficits included support (both emotional and organisational) to the dying and their families, communication, symptom management, and family-centred decision making, which they suggested concurs with the current evidence regarding what people want from end of life care to facilitate a 'good death'. In addition, they identified the difficulties inherent in describing what a good death should be. This should continue to be of concern because although there is a drive to support people to die in their home environment, there are still a considerable number of people who require hospital admission at the end of life due to unresolved symptoms or other unforeseen conditions, as well as some desire to be nursed in what they perceive as a 'safe' environment (Age Concern 2008).

## The predictability of death

Many older people may detect when death is near but still have similar fears and concerns regarding what that may bring or what they may expect (Ridgeway 2011). Being prepared and having time to discuss their anxieties may help to alleviate these concerns. There are similarities when nursing younger patients with a progressive, life-limiting illness. It will also be challenging and may involve caring for a distressed family unit who need support and information besides a number of key interventions and additional services (Humphreys and Rose 2011). In all cases, identifying when death is approaching may help to prepare for the inevitable and give the opportunity to say goodbye to their loved ones.

To address the issues surrounding the timing and predictability of death, the Gold Standards Framework (Thomas 2011) introduced a prognostic indicator tool (see Chapter 9 for further discussion). The aim is to aid in the identification of those nearing end of life, but it does not help to differentiate between hours, days, weeks or months. This tool is a useful resource to help identify when discussions surrounding end of life care should be initiated; in addition to this, one may need to identify those who are in the last few hours or days of life rather than simply the last few weeks or months. These distinctions may require other indicators. NICE (2015) announced a draft of their impending guidance surrounding caring for the dying adult and one of the recommendations aims to help identify those nearing end of life which may be helpful for health and social care staff. The expected release of the full guidance is December 2015. As one becomes more experienced, what some refer to as a 'gut instinct' can help to predict when time is short. Although gut instinct insinuates a subjective and less scientific approach, it may be that it is based upon previous experience and reflection (Benner 1984).

### Case scenario: James

James, aged 66, had been diagnosed with bowel cancer for 4 years. He had surgery and subsequent chemotherapy. His bowel cancer had spread to his liver and further investigations revealed it was inoperable. James deteriorated rapidly and became withdrawn. He felt he could not really speak to his wife, and all the family appeared to be getting on with their life. His appetite decreased substantially and he stopped eating with his family. He had lost over half his body weight and he was extremely fatigued. He was admitted to the hospital with vomiting and he had significant pain which scored 8 out of 10 on the pain assessment tool. He was currently taking the maximum dose of co-codamol with no effect. He was seen by the consultant and after further investigation they found he was in sub-acute obstruction (partial bowel obstruction). His condition deteriorated and he was unable to eat and became extremely lethargic, sleeping most of the time. He could not drink so the nursing staff provided him with regular mouthcare.

## Reflection points

- What are the signs and symptoms that would indicate James is dying?
- What would you need to put in his care plan?
- What would you need to discuss with James?
- What about his family?
- Think about James' pain; how would you describe it?

Expertise and experience do help to identify when a patient is dying by acknowledging signs and symptoms which may well indicate that time is limited, but this can still present even the most experienced with a challenge at times (Baldwin and Woodhouse 2011; Chapman and Ellershaw 2011). Rather than dwelling on the length of time, Twycross and Wilcock (2001) state that giving appropriate treatment is vital to ensure that symptoms are managed effectively. Assessing the patient as they approach the terminal phase of illness is vital to determine the appropriateness of any interventions and treatments (Chapman and Ellershaw 2011). In addition, ongoing assessment, monitoring and evaluation are crucial as patients deteriorate, paying attention to detail in order to prevent unnecessary patient suffering. Communication between all concerned is also essential in order to ensure continuity and preparedness for what the future holds (NICE 2015). Ensuring that James receives appropriate and effective pain relief is vital, and oral agents should be avoided in this case due to his vomiting: he may not be absorbing anything he takes orally, therefore leaving him with unresolved symptoms. Parental drug administration via a portable syringe driver would be helpful in delivering James' treatment as he requires opiate analgesia and an anti-emetic medication. This is delivered as a continuous subcutaneous infusion and can provide a safe and effective means of administering a number of drugs at the same time. Delivering the anti-emetic in this way should have a good effect due to its guaranteed absorption, and the analgesia, by administering over a constant infusion, will eradicate the peaks and troughs associated with regular injections of opiates or administration of oral preparations (Twycross and Wilcock 2001; British National Formulary 2014).

 ## Case scenario: Tom

Tom is 18 and was diagnosed with sarcoma. He was receiving palliative treatment as his curative therapy had failed. He and his family attended clinic to see when his next treatment would be. He was seen by the oncologist and the Macmillan nurse. Following a long and difficult discussion they had been informed that there was no further treatment and that they would adopt supportive measures, which meant that they would try to keep him comfortable and symptom free. He discussed his concerns and fears, but also managed to talk about what he wanted. This was to remain at home and to have his friends and family around him at the end of life. The palliative care team with the district nurse, GP and social worker managed to support the family and Tom right up to the day he died. He died peacefully listening to his favourite music and had managed to speak to his friends shortly before his death.

## Reflection points

Think about Tom's death:

- How would this fit with your ideas of a good death?
- If you had been nursing Tom, how would you feel having contributed to his end of life care?
- How do you think his family would feel after his death?

Although grief is a distressing experience where one has to come to terms with the loss of a loved one, knowing that they were cared for exactly as they had wished and had excellent support with effective symptom management may help to ease the pain of grief. This would make sense when one examines some of the criteria (see Figure 10.1) identified within the literature surrounding what a good death should include: having control over pain and other symptom relief (Age Concern 2008); dying in their chosen place (Miyashita et al. 2008); good relationship with family (Miyashita et al. 2015); knowledge and expertise of the staff caring and supporting those requiring end of life care and their loved ones (Cagle et al. 2015).

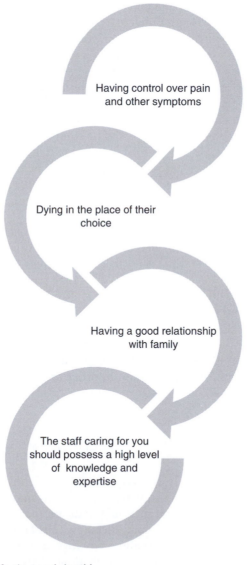

**Figure 10.1**   Criteria for 'a good death'

Adapted from Cagle et al. (2015)

A good death can be considered a positive experience from a number of perspectives. For a patient with a life-limiting illness, the reassurance that they will not suffer or be afraid may help them to live the remainder of their life more peacefully, without fearing the death itself. For their loved ones, seeing them die pain free and peacefully may be comforting and leave a sense of knowing that everyone has done their best. For staff caring for them, they may feel they have done the best for their patient and feel a sense of achievement that they were able to respect the patient's wishes, achieving good symptomatic control.

There are a number of beliefs and perceptions surrounding what one may believe a good death to be, and although individuals have ideas about symptom relief and so on, a comprehensive explanation or description evades us as the participants in Cipolletta and Oprandi's study (2014) demonstrated when asked what they thought a good death was. Although the researchers suggested that the difficulties may be due to the discomfort associated with care of the dying, it may also be due to the individuality and beliefs of those caring for the dying. As individuals we have our own beliefs and wishes surrounding what we would want or not want, therefore to have one idealistic description or tick list to complete for a good death may be unrealistic. If it was as simple as this, then attempting to ascertain what people want at the end of life would not be necessary as it would all be the same. This reinforces the importance of communication at the end of life and determining people's wishes in order to try to promote a good death. One may suggest that a good death should include a patient's last wishes, whenever possible.

As already established, a good death is what we aim to achieve when delivering palliative and end of life care, but one must be mindful of the fact that staff providing end of life care, over time, may become distressed themselves and have inadequate time for debrief and reflection. This may have a detrimental effect on their own health and wellbeing (see Chapter 11). Whilst striving to provide a good death we need time and space to express our own needs, so although one may feel positive in the belief that Tom died in the manner he wished once he was aware that there was no further treatment for his primary disease, the impact of nursing a patient to the end of life may still affect us personally over time. Consequently, we need to learn to care for ourselves too in order to continue to deliver the same high standard of care to all.

## Indicators that death is approaching

Identifying when a patient is dying may be helped by looking for more specific symptoms and patient presentations, which in isolation may suggest very little but if a number of them are identified, they may indicate that the patient or client is, indeed, in the dying phase. Chapman and Ellershaw (2011) suggested that the multidisciplinary team agreement surrounding whether a patient is dying is more important and accurate than clinical indicators alone. This statement advocates for effective interprofessional working to help identify those nearing end of life and to prepare them as much as possible. Nurses should still try to use their assessment skills, however, to alert the team to the possibilities regarding patients in their care and the stage they are in their illness.

Signs and symptoms which may be displayed as a patient approaches end of life include changes in breathing pattern, inability to eat and drink, and more obviously, unconsciousness and an unresponsive state. Other subtle indicators may be changes in skin colour and texture (patient's skin may take on a 'waxy' appearance and become pale) as the organs begin to fail, urine output may diminish and there may be a reduction of circulating blood to the peripheries (i.e. fingers and toes, giving a blue/purple, mottled appearance). If a patient is being given comfort care only and deemed to be in the terminal phase of illness, investigations like blood testing and routine observations may be stopped, therefore those clinical indicators that we generally use to warn of a deteriorating condition cannot help in identifying when death is imminent. Effective assessment can help in the care of these patients and ensure that prompt proactive care is delivered, but also allows us to keep relatives and loved ones informed of the current condition and gives an opportunity to guide and support them through the experience rather than leaving them isolated and fearful. How people die remains in the memory of those who live on, which includes relatives, carers, health and social care staff and so on (DH 2008).

## Reflection points

Think about any patients you may have looked after at the end of life:

- Can you recognise any of these signs?
- Did they have any symptoms that you had to give some treatment for?
- How did you support their relatives and/or carers?

Symptom management at the end of life may present challenges. It is important to remember that not all patients have pain, nausea or excessive secretions, for example. If symptoms are present and a patient has not refused specific treatments, then it is the healthcare team's responsibility to ensure that the patient does not suffer and be left untreated and neglected (General Medical Council 2010; NMC 2015).

The holistic assessment of James, earlier in this chapter, was vital. His pain was multidimensional and he was clearly suffering physically as well as psychologically, socially, emotionally and spiritually. Saunders (1963b) suggested the theory of total pain, where it encompassed all these elements for patients with advancing disease. There is a clear distinction between acute pain, which has a beginning, an end and a reason, from chronic pain or that associated with advancing illness where no end can be seen (Saunders and Baines 1984) other than in death itself and, as it involves the whole person, it is overwhelming and threatening to the individuality of that person as it consumes their existence.

## Reflection point

- Read this piece of narrative about death and dying and reflect on your experience:

  The spirituality of those who care for the dying must be the spirituality of the companion, of the friend who walks alongside, helping, sharing and sometimes just sitting, empty handed, when one would rather run away. It is the spirituality of *presence*, of being alongside, watchful, available, of being there. (Cassidy 1988, cited by Watson et al. 2009: 753)

Being 'available' for guidance, support and helping is vital as a person reaches the end of life (Twycross and Wilcock 2001). The patient should be able to discuss their wishes and concerns, anxieties and beliefs without fear of being judged. Support is also vital for their partners and loved ones as they embark on an unwanted journey where fear, anxiety and distress may dominate.

## Symptom management at the end of life

### Pain

Pain is often associated with deteriorating illness and requires a comprehensive approach in its assessment to ensure that a holistic approach is adopted. Stringent documentation regarding any interventions, including the effectiveness, is paramount so that repeated use of ineffective therapies is prevented and thereby patient suffering is avoided. The Parliamentary and Health Service Ombudsman (2015) uncovered reports of patients being left in pain as they reached the end of life. Every available resource should be utilised until the patient can be deemed pain free. Although this may be a difficult challenge, to not do anything is unforgivable and breaches ethical, moral and professional codes (NMC 2015).

Pain relief is selected via the World Health Organization's analgesic ladder (2004) (see Chapter 9 regarding end of life care planning). What one must consider when discussing pain relief with a patient and staff is the patient's current analgesic requirements, their anticipated future needs, and the current condition and its predicted pathway (i.e. the potential need for rescue medication – medication prescribed in anticipation of their deterioration). One needs to be mindful that the patient's psychological, emotional, spiritual and social distress relating to their pain should also be assessed, as pain relief will not address these concerns. Saunders (1963a) suggested that psychological pain is the most difficult pain to treat and alleviate.

## Case scenario: Joan

Joan, aged 74, has oesophageal carcinoma. She has lost a great deal of weight and she has some right flank pain and epigastric discomfort. She has been taking co-codamol regularly but this has not resolved her pain completely and she has severe pain before her next dose is due. A recent ultrasound has indicated the presence of multiple liver metastases. Joan is now struggling to swallow food and her weight loss is significant.

## Reflection points

- What are your concerns about Joan and her pain relief?
- What do you need to do?
- What are your options regarding her pain relief?
- What discussions should be taking place with Joan?

Joan's prognosis is poor and her difficulties with swallowing will only get worse. The tumour is invading her oesophagus and the likelihood is that she will occlude completely. In addition, the liver metastases are causing some pain, which will need to be considered when deciding on pain relief because many opiates need a reasonable liver function to excrete them, and blood tests to determine albumin levels and clotting times are good measures of function. If this is poor the opiates may not be completely cleared, leaving increasing levels of opiate as each dose is administered. This is similar in renal impairment, where the effects of opiates are increased and prolonged (British National Formulary 2014). The patient should be assessed regularly regarding their analgesic needs using a holistic philosophy as their comfort is the priority rather than any concerns about the dose of analgesia they require. Joan needs to be aware of the fact that she may get to the point where she cannot swallow, so discussion surrounding feeding may need initiating. Currently her pain relief is ineffective as she has residual discomfort as well as severe pain before her next dose is due. Experiencing a recurrence of pain before the next dose may be termed 'pre-dose breakthrough' and could suggest the need for a higher dose. What is certain is that to ignore this pain would be bad practice (Twycross and Wilcock 2001).

# Nutrition and hydration

Clinically assisted nutrition and hydration at the end of life is a significant ethical and moral issue which may leave us feeling anxious about whether it should be initiated or not. We may be anxious about whether it is facilitating relief or incurring further suffering. The National Council for Palliative Care (2007) produced guidance to try to demystify and clarify the issues within this dilemma, but suggested that patient assessment was paramount as it may be appropriate to initiate in some but not all cases. A further audit by the Royal College of Physicians (2014) still identified failures in communicating and discussing clinically assisted nutrition and hydration at the end of life with the patients themselves or their relatives if they are unable. In addition, documenting discussions and providing mouthcare when oral intake has ceased still need attention. The guidelines from NICE (2015) aim to give further advice when considering hydration at the end of life but also reiterate the importance of mouthcare when patients start to refuse oral fluids or are incapable of taking fluids orally.

What is evident is that clinically assisted hydration at the end of life can increase the fluid load within the body, and when organs are failing it may result in oedema and a build-up of respiratory secretions. Both these effects may be distressing to the patient and/or the relatives as well as the staff caring for them (De Souza 2013) (see Chapters 8 and 9 regarding clinically assisted hydration at the end of life).

The Royal College of Physicians (2014) identified that there continues to be a large number of deaths that occur in hospital, and there needs to be a significant improvement in the communication and decision making for patients as they reach the end of life. In the case note audit, 45 per cent of patients were assessed for clinically assisted nutrition (CAN) and hydration (CAH), but only 17 per cent of those had been discussed with the patient themselves and 29 per cent had been discussed with the family. Only 7 per cent of patients had CAN or CAH in place at the time of their death. The audit suggested that decisions such as the use of CAH and CAN should be made by senior, experienced clinicians and the multidisciplinary team, but that it should also be discussed with the patient when possible and include the carers or relatives if applicable. There are times when CAH may be useful in helping to relieve distressing symptoms, but one needs to ensure that the patient is well enough to undertake the artificial fluid load and the body able to use it to treat the symptom or condition for which it is being initiated (e.g. urinary tract infection or dry mouth) (De Souza 2013).

# Dignity in death, how to facilitate it

Dignity is a human right and to deprive someone of their dignity may be punishable in law (Human Rights Act 1998). The NMC states that as a registered nurse a person's human rights must be respected and upheld whilst treating them with 'kindness and compassion' (NMC 2015: 4). The Royal College of Nursing introduced the *Dignity at the Heart of Everything We Do* campaign in 2008–9. They identified that dignity is fundamental to everything we do and deprivation of dignity can manifest in a number of ways, but the ultimate effect is one of distress and may result in atrocities such as those seen at Mid Staffordshire (DH 2013a) or Winterbourne (DH 2013b). They identified through their research what dignity meant to individuals: it was a feeling of self-worth and a valuing of others. Therefore, in contrast, to deprive someone of their dignity would be to devalue them and incite feelings of worthlessness.

Relating these definitions to palliative care, when a patient approaches the end of life and loses their ability to function normally, including perhaps some loss of their spiritual self, then to add to this a deprivation of dignity, their life may become unbearable. The BBC *Panorama* programme 'Behind Closed Doors' (2014) identified scenes of abuse, assault and inadequate care within a nursing home, and showed there was little evidence of people's dignity being considered or maintained in the caring environment. Being left in soiled sheets or pads, being knowingly left needing the toilet, deliberate removal of the client's call bell are just a few examples of what may be perceived as deprivation of dignity. As the Royal College of Nursing (2008) suggests, dignity may be reinforced by good care or it may be eradicated with poor care, and both these scenarios can be achieved through the attitudes and behaviours of staff, the environment, the culture of the organisation facilitating the care or the care itself and the way it is delivered.

For the patient who is reaching the end of life, not having their needs met (e.g. inadequate acknowledgement of symptom burden, being left for long periods leading to feelings of isolation, poor communication between the team and the patient) may threaten a patient's dignity. Once again, comprehensive, ongoing, assessment and monitoring can help to indicate any symptom burden and identify distress. Ensuring that responsive and proactive care is delivered in line with the patient's needs and wishes may help to maintain a patient's dignity. Communication needs to be effective and understandable. It should also be delivered at a pace appropriate to the patient and their carers or relatives. This should facilitate a patient-centred approach (see Chapter 7 regarding the importance of communication).

## Reflection points

Examine once again the carer's narrative at the end of Chapter 5 (pp. 67–73):

- In what ways do you think Emily's dignity was deprived whilst in hospital?
- How did this change when Emily was at home being nursed by her daughters?

Being deprived of pain relief does not necessarily mean having none at all, but stating to a patient who is in pain, 'You have had all your prescribed pain relief so you will have to wait until the next dose is due' is depriving someone of their basic right to be free of pain. The nurse should offer their support and get the analgesic regime reviewed in order to ensure that prescribed pain relief is adequate and meets the patient's current analgesic requirements.

A dignified death can help those left behind in their grief. What constitutes a dignified death may be quite individual, similarly to what constitutes a good death. Once again, there may be some commonalities; it may be rare that one wants to suffer excruciating pain to the end but that does not mean it would never happen. In many cases, if loved ones witness a peaceful death where the dying appeared to be calm, pain free and comfortable, then despite the ensuing pain associated with the loss it may be more bearable than if they had witnessed intense suffering or obvious distress, but again this would depend on individual beliefs. A distressing death may leave relatives feeling disempowered and useless as they could not induce any positive influence over the last days of life to minimise their loved one's suffering. The daughters in the Chapter 5 case scenario exerted their influence, and through their wishes to meet their mother's needs – and to some extent their own, which was wanting to do one selfless act and care for their mum in a loving environment until she died – they managed to preserve Emily's dignity and witness her peaceful death together. This could have been very different had her syringe driver not been initiated and the services not been in place. In addition, the perseverance of Emily's daughters to try to ensure that their mum was supported and should not feel afraid again was a driving force that helped their mum achieve a peaceful, dignified death.

## Grief models

There are a number of models to help and assist people through their grief and bereavement. Kubler Ross (1970) is well known for her stages of grief and the suggestion that the individual should 'move' through the stages, from denial at the death through to the final stage of acceptance. This suggestion of acceptance perhaps carries the most conflict, with many theorists and researchers suggesting that this is unachievable in many instances (Stroebe and Schut 1999) and some arguing that other feelings may be more pertinent when dealing with loss, such as gratitude or wisdom, which Redwood (2002) proposes may have a more spiritual meaning to loss. Mallon (2008) highlights that a number of variables influence the way in which people grieve (e.g. culture and religion), but one may also suggest that past experiences and situations may also have a profound effect on the way a person grieves or displays their grief.

Other grief theories revolve around identifying it as 'normal', and if not normal then it must be 'delayed,' 'absent' or 'chronic' (Wortman and Silver 2001), and Worden (1991) suggests 'relocating the deceased into your new life' rather than trying to forget them. The work of Stroebe and Schut (1999) was quite different in that they moved away from stages and a linear movement through a process. This was replaced with the idea that people revolve between 'loss orientated coping' to 'restorative orientated coping'. This broadly means missing their loved one and dwelling on the loss, then moving to a more optimistic position, thinking about the future and getting on with life or the issues at hand. Thinking about their loved one and dealing with that loss is fixed within loss orientate coping, whilst the restorative oriented coping is the individual's attempt to continue with life. There is an understanding that the person may orientate between the two domains interchangeably and challenges may present which results in them moving into the loss orientated phase (e.g. a shared experience, birthdays, special occasions where the loved one is missing). Trying to build a life without the loved one physically sharing it may be difficult, therefore the movement between loss and restorative domains would appear to be a rational way to view the bereavement experience.

## Case scenario: Linda

Linda, aged 35, lost her husband John 6 months ago. He died following a short illness. She has two children, Harvey and Beth, whom she feels very grateful for as they are a constant reminder of the life she shared with him. Her life has obviously changed dramatically over the last 6 months, but she realised after the first few weeks that she still has two children and a life to lead. She decides to apply for a new job so that she has a fresh start. It was difficult as everyone knew about John in her current employment. She is lucky enough to find new employment and she starts to spend more quality time with the children. They start new activities together, such as indoor climbing, and she feels that although she still misses John she has to live for both of them and for the children.

It was Harvey's birthday and although Linda manages to organise and give him a fun day, at bedtime she feels exhausted and overwhelmed. She cries for what feels like hours and struggles to think of a life without John. The next morning she gets up and makes breakfast and prepares for another day. Eventually she feels a little more positive about the future and what it may hold.

## Reflection points

- Can you make sense of Linda's emotional rollercoaster?
- Can you identify which grief model best fits her experience?
- What do you think of Linda's responses?

Grief is a very personal experience and although we may be able to identify key characteristics and label some of the cognitive experiences which 'fit' with some of the theories, it is important to remember the person who is experiencing the grief. Trying to determine where they are in the grief cycle may not be of any use to the grieving person, but determining whether their grief is overwhelming and consuming to the point that you are concerned that it is enduring for a protracted length of time, or that it is having detrimental physical effects on the individual, is a more important factor to identify.

## Complex bereavement

Complex grief may present in many ways but has been identified as delayed or an incomplete adaption to their loss (Payne et al. 1999). It is important to be familiar with some of the 'triggers' which have been associated with a risk of complex bereavement in order to act in a more responsive manner or provide greater support to an individual deemed at risk.

A significant amount of research has been undertaken in order to identify some of the triggers to incomplete or complex bereavement (Parkes and Weiss 1983; Kushner 1982; Shear et al. 2005; Ribbens McCarthy 2005; Elliot 1999; Blackman 2008). A number of situations or circumstances have been proposed. These include: sudden death; death which occurred whilst there was ongoing hostility or unresolved situations; when the bereaved had some psychological traits or issues which led then to a vulnerable state; recurrent or multiple losses; and those who are, or feel, isolated.

## Reflection points

- Think about the triggers identified that could lead to an incomplete or complex bereavement pattern.
- Identify the reasons why these situations could ensue the complex bereavement circumstances discussed.

Many of the causes or contributors in unresolved or difficult bereavement experiences may derive from the lack of a 'good death'. We have already established that a good death should be recognised as the gold standard management of those reaching the end of life. This constitutes a number of perceptions and emotions, which may include: a chance to say goodbye; effective symptom management of psychological, social and spiritual issues; and a patient-centred approach which involves empowering the individual as they approach the end of life, giving them a chance or opportunity to discuss their wishes for their own end of life care.

## Reflection points

- Think again about what may constitute a good death.
- What would you want?
- What issues could there be that puts a good death at risk?

Care of the patient as they are approaching death is a time where excellent nursing care is particularly vital. Ensuring patient comfort and freedom from distressing symptoms can mean the patient dies peacefully, which for a loved one, although they may be distressed at the loss, may allow them to reflect on the serenity of the death itself and be comforted by the fact that there was little or no perception of suffering.

## Conclusion

Dealing with the dying is an emotive experience where one may feel overwhelmed. Being able to provide effective, responsive, compassionate, dignified care to those at the end of life and support for their loved ones can help to give some satisfaction to those within the caring role. The *Consultation on Strengthening the NHS Constitution* (DH 2013c: 23) stated that 'treating everyone with dignity and respect' is paramount, and this wording was designed to emphasise the importance of dignity and respect. In addition, the latest NHS constitution states that 'Respect, dignity, compassion and care should be at the core of how patients ... are treated', which echoes again the previous guidance (NHS 2015:3).

Identifying when death may be imminent appears to be extremely important to the individual and to their loved ones. Ensuring your skills and knowledge about not only the identification of the indicators which may be present but also in symptom management and communication should be paramount in order to provide a high standard of care to the dying patient.

Anticipating complex grief reactions may help to signpost those at risk at an earlier stage so that effective support and treatment may be given. Supporting the individual through their own grief and recognising that grief models are not meant to be prescriptive should be acknowledged, as they can to help identify where additional support may be required.

Dealing with the dying is a privilege, and one should not be reticent of the impact that high-quality care can have on the journey of not only the patient but also their loved ones.

## Reflection point

- Think again about the daughter's experience in the carer's narrative in Chapter 5 (pp. 67–73). If she had received greater support and more responsive care, then her grief may have been a little different.

## Recommended reading

Age Concern (2008) *Policy Position Papers: Dying and Death*. London: Age Concern.

Cagle, J.G., Pek, J., Clifford, M., Guralnik, J. and Zimmerman, S. (2015) 'Correlations of a good death and the impact of hospice involvement: Findings from the national survey of households affected by cancer', *Supportive Care Cancer*, 23: 809–18.

Chapman, L. and Ellershaw, J. (2011) 'Care in the last hours and days of life', *Medicine*, 39(11): 674–7.

## References

Age Concern (1999) *Debate of the Age, Health and Care Study Group: The Future of Health and Care of Older People: The Best is Yet to Come*. London: Age Concern.

Age Concern (2008) *Policy Position Papers: Dying and Death*. London: Age Concern.

Baldwin, M. and Woodhouse, J. (2011) *Key Concepts in Palliative Care*. London: Sage.

Benner, P. (1984) *From Novice to Expert: Excellence and Power in Clinical Practice*. Berkeley, CA: Addison Wesley.

Blackman, N. (2008) 'The development of an assessment tool for the bereaved needs of people with learning disabilities', *British Journal of Learning Disability*, 36(3): 165–70.

British Broadcasting Corporation (2014) *Behind Closed Doors*. London: BBC.

British National Formulary (2014) *British National Formulary (BNF) 68 (Sept. 2014 – March 2015)*. London: BMJ Group and Pharmaceutical Press.

Cagle, J.G., Pek, J., Clifford, M., Guralnik, J. and Zimmerman, S. (2015) 'Correlations of a good death and the impact of hospice involvement: Findings from the national survey of households affected by cancer', *Supportive Care Cancer*, 23: 809–18.

Cassidy, S. (1988) *Sharing the Darkness: The Spirituality of Caring*. London: Darton, Longman & Todd.

Chapman, L. and Ellershaw, J. (2011) 'Care in the last hours and days of life', *Medicine*, 39(11): 674–7.

Cialkowska-Rysz, A. and Dzierzanowski, T. (2013) 'Personal fear of death affects the proper process of breaking bad news', *Archives of Medical Science*, 9(1): 127–31.

Cipolletta, S. and Oprandi, N. (2014) 'What is a good death? Healthcare professionals' narrations on end of life care', *Death Studies*, 38: 20–7.

De Souza, J. (2013) 'Knowing when a patient is in the last days of life', in J. De Souza and A. Pettifer (eds), *End of Life Nursing Care*. London: Sage, pp. 124–40.

Department of Health (2008) *End of Life Care Strategy*. London: DH.

Department of Health (2013a) *Report of the Mid Staffordshire NHS Foundation Trust Public Enquiry.* London: DH.

Department of Health (2013b) *Transforming Care: A National Response to Winterbourne View Hospital.* London: DH.

Department of Health (2013c) *Consultation on Strengthening the NHS Constitution: Government Response.* London: DH.

Elliot, J.L. (1999) 'The death of a parent in childhood: A family account', *Illness Crisis and Loss,* 7(4): 360–75.

General Medical Council (2010) *Treatment Towards the End of Life: Good Practice in Decision Making.* Manchester: General Medical Council.

Human Rights Act (1998) *Chapter 42.* London: The Stationery Office.

Humphreys, A. and Rose, P. (2011) 'Caring for young people', in M. Baldwin and J. Woodhouse (eds), *Key Concepts in Palliative Care.* London: Sage, pp. 31–6.

Kubler Ross, E. (1970) *On Death and Dying.* London: Tavistock.

Kushner, H. (1982) *When Bad Things Happen to Good People.* London: Pan.

Mallon, B. (2008) *Dying, Death and Grief: Working with Adult Bereavement.* London: Sage

Miyashita, M., Kawakami, S., Kato, D., Yamashita, H., Igaki, H., Nakano, K., Kuroda, Y. and Nakagawa, K. (2015) 'The importance of good death components among cancer patients, the general population, oncologists, and oncology nurses in Japan: Patients prefer "fighting against cancer"', *Supportive Care Cancer,* 23: 103–10.

Miyashita, M., Morita T., Sato, K., Hirai, K., Shima, Y. and Uchitomi, Y. (2008) 'Good death inventory: A measure for evaluating good death from the bereaved family member's perspective', *Journal of Pain and Symptom* Management, 35(5): 486–98.

National Council for Palliative Care (2007) *Artificial Nutrition and Hydration: Guidance in End of Life Care for Adults.* London: NCPC.

National Health Service (2015) *The NHS Constitution: The NHS Belongs to US All.* London: NHS.

National Institute for Health and Care Excellence (2011) *CG121 Lung Cancer: The Diagnosis and Treatment of Lung Cancer.* London: NICE.

National Institute for Health and Care Excellence (2015) *Care of the Dying Adult: Guidance in Progress.* London: NICE. Available at: www.nice.org.uk/guidance/indevelopment/gid-cgwave0694. (accessed 20 August).

Nursing and Midwifery Council (2015) *The Code: Professional Standards of Practice and Behaviour for Nurses and Midwives.* London: NMC.

Parkes, C.M. and Weiss, R.S. (1983) *Recovery from Bereavement.* New York: Basic Books.

Parliamentary and Health Service Ombudsman (2015*) Dying without Dignity: Investigations by the Parliamentary and Health Service Ombudsman into Complaints about End of Life Care.* London: Parliamentary and Health Service Ombudsman.

Payne, S., Horn, S. and Relf, M. (1999) *Loss and Bereavement.* Buckingham: Open University Press.

Redwood, D. (2002) 'Dr Redwood interviews: Rachel Naomi Remen living in the post 9/11 world', cited by B. Mallon (2008), *Dying, Death and Grief: Working with Adult Bereavement.* London: Sage.

Ribbens McCarthy, J. (2005) 'The meaning of "meaning": Towards an inter-disciplinary and multi-method approach to bereavement'. Presentation at the *7th International Conference on Grief and Bereavement in Contemporary Society,* 12–15 July, Kings College, London.

Ridgeway, V. (2011) 'Caring for the older person', in M. Baldwin and J. Woodhouse (eds), *Key Concepts in Palliative Care.* London: Sage, pp. 26–30.

Royal College of Nursing (2008) *Dignity at the Heart of Everything We Do*. London: RCN.

Royal College of Physicians (2014) *National Care of the Dying Audit For Hospitals, England*. London: Royal College of Physicians.

Saunders, C. (1963a) 'The treatment of intractable pain in terminal cancer', *Proceedings of the Royal Society of Medicine*, 56(3): 195–7.

Saunders, C. (1963b) 'Care of the dying', *Current Medical Abstracts for Practitioners*, 3(2): 77–82.

Saunders, C. and Baines, M. (1984) *Living with Dying*. New York: Oxford University Press.

Shear, M.K., Frank, E., Houck, P.R. and Reynolds, C.F. (2005) 'Treatment of complicated grief: A randomised controlled trial', *Journal of American Medical Association*, 293: 2601–08.

Steinheuser, K.E., Christakis, N., Clipp, E.C., McNeilly, M., Mclntyre, L., and Tulsky, J.A. (2000) 'Factors considered important at the end of life by patients, family, physicians and other care providers', *Journal of the American Medical Association*, 28(19): 2476–82.

Stroebe, M. and Schut, H. (1999) 'The dual model of coping with bereavement: Rationale and description', *Death Studies*, 23: 197–224.

Thomas, K. (2011) *The GSF Prognostic Indicator Guidance: The National GSF Centre's Guidance for Clinicians to Support Earlier Recognition of Patients Nearing the End of Life*. Birmingham: Gold Standards Framework.

Twycross, R. and Wilcock, A. (2001) *Symptom Management in Advanced Cancer*, 3rd edn. Oxford: Radcliffe Medical Press.

Watson, M., Lucas, C., Hoy, A. and Wells, J. (2009) *Oxford Handbook of Palliative Care*, 2nd edn. Oxford: Oxford University Press.

Worden, J.W. (1991) *Grief Counselling and Grief Therapy: A Handbook for the Mental Health Practitioner*, 2nd edn. London: Routledge.

World Health Organization (2004) *Palliative Care and Symptom Management and End of Life Care: Integrated Management of Adolescent and Adult Illness*. Geneva: WHO.

Wortman, C.B. and Silver, R.C. (2001) 'The myths of coping with loss revisited', in M.S. Stroebe, R.O. Hansson, W. Stroebe and H. Schut (eds), *Handbook of Bereavement*. New York: Cambridge University Press. pp. 349–66.

# 11

# Support for the practitioner

## Martin Brock and Michelle Brown

---

This chapter will explore:

- stress and anxiety associated with palliative and end of life care for staff
- the nurse's role in care
- peer support
- compassion and self-compassion, and why it is important
- how to recognise your own needs
- the values and the impact on compassion
- some exercises to help 'the troubled self' and aid our wellbeing.

---

## Background

The Mid Staffordshire enquiry government response (Francis 2010) highlighted an abundance of failings with devastating consequences for patients, their families and loved ones. Jane Cummings introduced the 6 Cs (NHS 2012) as a means of re-establishing what nursing should embody, care attributes and behaviours that underpin nursing practice. The Nursing and Midwifery Council introduced more comprehensive requirements for pre-registration nurse education which involved clinical competency standards increasing from 17 within the four domains to 34 competencies (NMC 2010). The importance practice plays in the academic programme undertaken as education to degree level as a minimum was not devalued, but in fact the importance clinical practice plays in aiding student nurses to develop into competent practitioners is reiterated within those standards.

The experience and progression through a pre-registration programme may present challenges. End of life care is one specific aspect of nursing that has been highlighted in the NMC *Standards for Pre-registration Education* (2010). The Department of Health concurs with the NMC and suggests that end of life care education needs 'embedding in training curriculums at all levels and for all staff groups' (2010: 14) including student nurses. The Department of Health indicates, therefore, that the opportunity to gain further support and education is paramount for all staff members caring for patients at the end of life, not only to benefit patient care but also for the health and wellbeing of the staff involved.

## The nurse and their role in care

Lillyman et al. (2011) identified that the general population may not experience death until they themselves reach middle age, and those undertaking pre-registration nurse education may be no different to that. The average age of a person embarking on pre-registration nurse education may be reasonably young. The Royal College of Nursing (RCN) performed a survey in 2008 that indicated over half of those responding (53 per cent) were under 30 years old. 47 per cent of those who responded were over 30. Out of these, 17 per cent were between 35 and 40, and 19 per cent who were over 40. Over one-third of the participants in the UK were aged between 18 and 24 years (RCN 2008). This signifies the relevance of Lillyman et al.'s data regarding end of life experience, or rather the lack of it, amongst our pre-registration nursing student population, including those who have been accepted on the NMC register. Higher education institutions and employers may therefore have a significant number of students and newly qualified staff on their programmes or in post with little or no experience of death, yet within weeks of commencing their programme or employment they may be faced with the death of a patient and all the accompanying responsibilities.

During their practice placements, student nurses are assessed as nursing programmes are competency based (NMC 2010). Student nurses may view their own distress negatively as they perceive that other members of staff are 'dealing with death' and appear to be seemingly 'undisturbed'. Perhaps the belief that death is part of nursing may insinuate that one has to 'get on with it' and 'deal with it' as with any other aspects of care, and not getting 'emotionally involved' may incite barriers and cause the student to hide their distress and inhibit their desire to share or seek support. A recently qualified staff nurse may have a similar experience and fear being judged as 'weak' and 'incompetent' if they are seen to be 'upset' or 'distressed' when delivering palliative or end of life care.

## The student experience

Students may speak of 'feeling weak' and believe that they need to 'harden up emotionally', and many nurses have described distancing themselves from patients as a coping strategy (Mackintosh 2007). This may be a relatively common experience for student nurses and those who have recently qualified, but what one should ask is, 'Are these feelings appropriate?' Should we be affected by the gradual decline of another human being?

---

### Case scenario: Judy (part 1)

Judy, the student nurse we encountered in Chapter 7, was on her management placement. She was concerned that she had relatively no experience of caring for a patient at the end of life. She recalled her anxiety in year one when an elderly patient died but remembers the lack of concern from the staff members. She still feels that delivering end of life care will upset her. She is on a ward caring for people with respiratory disease and knows that delivering end of life care may be part of her role.

She speaks to her mentor about her anxieties as she has indicated this as a weakness on her SWOT analysis. Her mentor, Elizabeth, has been qualified for some time and appears perplexed regarding her concerns. Elizabeth states that it is part of the job and you have to get on with it because 'we have not got time to care for staff, we are too busy with patients!'

---

### Reflection points

- How does this scenario make you feel?
- Can you identify with some of Judy's concerns?
- What is Judy displaying by discussing it with her mentor?
- What is her mentor displaying in her response?
- How could Elizabeth have helped Judy?

---

Many staff members may be reluctant to share feelings for fear of being judged. The consequences of this could be harmful and may mean that staff begin to work in isolation and break team morale as there may be little support perceived by anyone. This could have a detrimental effect on patient care; as already established in earlier chapters, teamworking and collaboration are crucial to effective, high-quality patient care.

## Peer support

Peer support promotes a sense of 'family' (Campbell et al. 1994) and may in turn deliver a sense of security. A greater sense of sharing and caring with and for each other can also be gained from peer support. 'Offloading' may generally be seen as positive, and students with end of life care experience can support those with little experience, thereby caring for each other. In addition, qualified staff supporting other members of staff and encouraging a sharing and supportive environment should have a positive impact on staff morale and patient care. Not only would this support those with little experience, it may also allow those with greater experience to 'tell their stories', which one could suggest is cathartic in itself.

The one thing that is needed, however, is self-compassion. Without self-compassion one may question whether an individual can truly be compassionate with anyone else. Attributes of self-compassion and self-care awareness have been associated with compassionate practice to others (Gilbert 2009), and this makes sense given that compassion asks us to be vulnerable with the vulnerable (Schantz 2007). An individual may be lacking in self-compassion; that is, the ability to forgive oneself, to realise that we ourselves have needs and may struggle at times. We can punish ourselves for believing that anxiety and distress in clinical situations are signs of weakness.

Despite the fact that the quality of nursing care and the wellness of the nurse giving that care are interdependent (Maben et al. 2012), it has been shown that many nurses do not engage in self-care activities (McAllister and McKinnon 2009).

There may be perceptions amongst healthcare professionals that there are 'permitted' and 'not permitted' feelings that one should experience, which may lead to staff having aversions to experiences that may challenge those perceptions; for example, always getting upset if someone asks 'Am I dying nurse?'. They therefore evade those who have asked this to other members of staff or avoid the patient who appears to be deteriorating for fear of the question being posed. Cialkowska-Rysz and Dzierzanowski (2013) examined this phenomenon in physicians and found a complete aversion to breaking bad news due to the stress they feel it induces, and concerns about a patient's possible response to the bad news as well as the anxiety and burden of responsibility. This is clearly unhealthy as a nurse will have to remain on guard in order to remove themselves from any potential threats, like dealing with difficult questions from those with a life-limiting illness. More importantly, this could result in a distressed patient receiving substandard care or care that lacks compassion. Peters et al. (2013) examined staff anxiety surrounding dying and coping with death in palliative care and emergency department settings. Nurses working in palliative care had lower levels of anxiety about death, whilst staff working in the emergency department had lower coping skills and higher anxiety, inducing death avoidance. This fear prompts the withdrawal 'I avoid death at all costs' (2013: 156) from those who are dying, resulting in patients receiving suboptimal care at the end of life. Providing a pathway of support is essential in allowing both student and qualified health and social care professionals to process their feelings and identify ways of managing them, either by using self-compassion resources or acknowledging a need for more formal interventions. Increasing coping strategies and understanding our own fears may help to address some of these issues.

## Reflection points

Think again about Judy, the student nurse in the case scenario above:

- How do you think Judy will deal with difficult questions?
- How do you think Judy will feel caring for a dying patient?
- What impact could her mentor Elizabeth's feelings about emotions have on Judy's self-compassion and compassion to others long term?

Judy may well care for a dying patient during this placement or any of the placements which follow, but her anxieties may provide her with obstacles in dealing with the situation. She may draw on her own inner resources and provide excellent end of life care which she reflects upon, and this could give her a sense of achievement and self-belief. The alternative is that she could be extremely distressed in dealing with the patient's demise and 'hold on to her feelings' because she feels that there is no time for emotions on the ward and feels weak in her inability to deal with it in what she perceives as a 'normal' way.

## Self-compassion

Van der Cingel (2014: 1254) identifies the strong links between compassion and high-quality care and describes it as an 'empowering characteristic' rather than 'a personal quality'. Given the fact that end of life care demands high-quality provision and delivery, compassion is vital from each health and social care professional who may be involved in that particular patient's journey. Poor-quality care is something that cannot be remedied at a later date; for the patient it may mean an undignified or difficult death, and for the relatives it may mean a complex bereavement experience fuelled by anger and regret as a result of poor care for their loved one. To be compassionate to others, however, there is a suggestion that one needs to be compassionate with oneself (Gilbert 2009).

 ## Case scenario: Ray

Ray, aged 73, was diagnosed with advanced heart failure and was fully aware of his prognosis along with his wife Hilda. Ray wanted to be nursed at home, but also wanted to feel that his symptoms were being addressed. As Ray was becoming more

*(Continued)*

(Continued)

symptomatic, his GP referred him to the district nursing team. The team were facing a number of challenges and there was little cohesion due to staff leaving and changes in sites. The district nurse visited on two occasions but both Ray and Hilda did not feel he was listened to. He was struggling with breathlessness and chest pain. The district nurse did not suggest any medication and the couple felt isolated. Ray died in pain and Hilda was overwhelmed not just with grief but also anger at their situation.

## Reflection points

- Can you empathise with Ray and Hilda's situation?
- What do you think the issues were for the district nurse?
- Do you feel the district nurse adopted a compassionate approach?
- What impact could Hilda's experience have on her bereavement?
- What could have happened for the district nurse to practice this way?
- What would you do to help this district nurse?

Patients with a non-cancer diagnosis are less likely to receive specialist palliative care input, which may be due to traditional views regarding it being predominantly for care of those with cancer (DH 2008). In the above case scenario, lack of input regarding symptom management for Ray and support for Hilda resulted in a significantly poor experience for both, and perhaps also for the district nurse and GP. Ray and Hilda wanted to be listened to and treated with compassion and dignity; this does not require a specialist team. The district nurse was clearly in a difficult situation with what appears to have very little peer support, and one may go further and suggest that what she was experiencing appeared to be quite the opposite of what she needed from her colleagues. Long-term this may have a significant impact on the district nurse and her ability to function in her role, but the impact for the patients in her care will be immeasurable. The aim of this scenario was to demonstrate the potential impact of not recognising your own needs and the consequences of failing to gain support from colleagues. The district nurse failed to recognise or respond to the suffering of others. One may argue that people need to feel they are listened to and that their 'total' pain (Saunders 1976) is acknowledged as this may provide them with some comfort. In this situation, however, not only did Ray and Hilda feel that death was traumatic, but the isolation and their traumatic experience was unrecognised.

# Recognising your own needs

There appears to be an overwhelming lack of self-compassion amongst healthcare professionals, culminating in feelings of shame and resulting in burnout (Irving et al. 2009). Self-critical and self-sacrificing attitudes were identified in physicians (Miller and McGowan 2000), but one may argue that this is endemic within healthcare generally as professional training has been identified as stressful due to managing academic requirements and balancing this with the stress and anxieties of clinical practice (Curtis et al. 2012), as well as the need to 'be helpful' when patients are in distress (Chandler et al. 2001). For the recently qualified nurse or other healthcare or social care professional, the need to establish credibility and be seen as fit for purpose and competent may generate similar stress and anxiety. There is a plethora of research surrounding role transition and the anxiety and feelings of uncertainty and inadequacy that this generates amongst a vast proportion of recently qualified staff, demonstrating that these are not isolated incidences (Higgins et al. 2010; Whitehead et al. 2013; Clark and Holmes 2007).

A particular area of concern is when healthcare professionals begin to feel isolated, for example: 'when I am feeling down I tend to obsess and fixate on everything that is wrong', which may have been one of the issues faced by the district nurse in the latter scenario.

## Case scenario: Judy (part 2)

Judy the student nurse continues to feel anxious about end of life care. She is allocated a bay of patients as part of her management responsibilities for completing her nursing programme. One of the patients has been diagnosed with lung cancer. This is a new diagnosis and Judy feels extremely apprehensive. The gentleman is 47 and she can't help but think about her partner who is only a little younger than this man. She is aware that he is dyspnoeic and he has had some haemoptysis recently, which has been treated with medication. Judy greets him and informs him that she will be looking after him today. When asked about hygiene care and so forth, he asks if she can help him as he feels exhausted and it exacerbates his breathlessness. She agrees to help and prepares all her equipment. As she helps him wash he breaks down crying and confides in her. He relays his anxieties about dying and leaving his wife and children behind. She becomes tearful and feels that she cannot deal with this. She cuts off the conversation and says she will be back shortly as she has forgotten something.

Once she feels she has 'pulled herself together' she returns to the task in hand and does not refer back to the conversation. He does not mention anything again either. When Judy finishes her shift she goes home and cries but is unsure what to do. She feels stupid and weak. She knows other people can manage these situations and feels a failure. She feels that perhaps nursing is not for her as she is too emotional.

## Reflection points

- Do you feel that Judy's crying was reasonable, given the situation?
- Is there any way she could have handled it better?
- Do you feel that Judy's thoughts once she finished her shift are rational?
- Have you ever had similar thoughts after a difficult shift?
- Is there any comparison between the advice you would give to Judy and that which you gave to yourself?

Nurses may ruminate and worry, and this suggests that they may have some self-blame for situations, shame and predict that others are handling things better than they are. Again, the student may experience this and perceive showing emotions to be a weakness and lack of competency and therefore may fear failure within the practice placement. The fixation surrounding what has gone wrong and tending to try to address it in isolation may result in the student withdrawing due to feeling that their competency may once again be questioned.

Consider for a moment this kind of reflection on oneself: 'I should have done better …', 'I must be stronger …', 'It is weak to let my feelings get in the way'.

Let us unpack this a little more from another perspective, that is, from our usual reactions to others in distress in the following exercise.

EXERCISE

## ↻ Understanding self-criticism

Find a quiet spot for yourself, perhaps a favourite armchair, and begin by settling yourself into this place.

Imagine for a moment that a friend had contacted you to talk about a slight mistake or error at work that was troubling them, and you had agreed to meet.

Your friend describes committing a rather minor error and it is clear that working long hours, with reduced staff and in a particularly busy and stressful working environment are contributing factors. Yet your friend describes a lot of shame and the sense of letting people down that has led to a number of self-criticisms:

'I should have done better, … I must be stronger … It is weak to let my feelings get in the way … I feel so stupid … I just don't think nursing is for me.'

## Reflection points

- How would you respond to your friend?
- Notice your reactions – what feelings and urges show up?

- What would you say to your friend and how would you say it? Notice the tone of voice and the language that you use.
- What are you trying to convey to your friend?
- Did you notice a lack of negative evaluation and criticism in your dialogue?
- Can you notice the 'kindness' evident in your responses and reactions?

In the scenario presented earlier, Judy felt she had handled the situation badly and that displaying her vulnerability and being emotionally affected by this situation demonstrated lack of competence, whereas one may argue being emotionally congruent with the suffering of her patient is an indicator of compassion and validation. This may signify the importance that self-compassion should have in nursing curriculums, higher education institutions and other staff development opportunities. Preparing employees for practice not just physically but also emotionally and psychologically, due to the demands that nursing may have on the workforce in both these domains, could have a positive effect on staff wellbeing and patient care.

## Compassion in education

What one may suggest is that a safe learning environment underpinned by a philosophy of 'shared compassion for all' may be beneficial to the health and wellbeing of the students as well as to their colleagues and the patients they will care for in the future. One should acknowledge that end of life care is a major part of the nursing role, and there needs to be an increased recognition regarding the importance of preparing healthcare professionals for this vital but potentially distressing responsibility.

Van der Cingel (2014) has called for compassion being integrated within nursing programmes. One may also suggest that in view of the theories surrounding self-compassion and its positive links with an ability to deliver compassionate care (Gilbert 2009), self-compassion should be a key part of nursing curricula. An example of how to achieve this has been shown by Gustin and Wagner (2013). If educational initiatives are developed that embody mindfulness practice, self-compassion training, values clarification and reflection on clinical experience, it should promote a culture for change. This should not only be located in pre-registration education but also run alongside mandatory training in practice areas. The introduction should improve end of life care experience not only for the staff, but also for patients and their loved ones as they will be cared for by healthcare professionals who have been supported and who feel prepared for the demands associated with end of life care provision both personally and professionally. Although this should improve care for those with non-life-limiting disease and illness, end of life care experiences specifically need processing as for any other distressing experience. By not processing it the distress can grow, resulting in an intensity which may cease to be manageable. Now look at the situation from your own perspective in the following exercise.

## ↻ Making your own mistakes

Now see if you can imagine that it was you yourself who had made this error or mistake and that it was you that 'felt stupid', 'should be stronger', 'should not let your feelings get in the way'.

---

## Reflection points

Notice your reactions:

- What feelings and urges show up?
- What would you say to yourself and how would you say it? Notice the tone of voice and the language you use.
- What are you trying to convey to yourself?
- Is this different from the way you reacted to your friend's distress?
- Consider the tone of this self-dialogue; what are we saying to ourselves, and how are we judging and evaluating our human reactions?
- Can you see how berating and punitive this can sound?

---

It is rather like suffering twice over; the experience of working in an emotionally demanding environment such as end of life care is taxing enough on our resources and yet we heap more emotional distress on ourselves by being critical and evaluating ourselves in a negative manner. Is it any wonder that professionals and carers working in end of life care report exhaustion and fatigue and that it is viewed as one of the most demanding of nursing roles (Hopkinson et al. 2005)?

Generally, people find that they are moved by another's suffering and show understanding, and empathy, and are comforting, hopeful and kind in their responses, and yet are more critical and negative when considering their own perceived transgressions (Neff 2003). In fact, it is often the case that extremely kind and compassionate people are incredibly harsh on themselves (Germer and Neff 2013). So, whilst this is not unusual, it is key to recognising our own emotional needs, particularly in healthcare as nurses may be tougher and less forgiving of themselves, which could make an already difficult healthcare experience harder to process and manage (Heffernan et al. 2010).

Returning to the key components of compassion (Dalai Lama 2002):

1. Being aware and recognising the suffering in others and self.
2. Engaging in and being moved by the suffering in others and self.
3. Acting to alleviate the suffering in others and self.

The key in terms of promoting our own wellbeing is developing awareness of our own suffering and the willingness to engage in and alleviate our own suffering. In essence, turning compassion towards ourselves and thus developing self-compassion (Neff 2010). Self-compassion can be useful when we find ourselves bogged down by self-criticism of our human flaws and mistakes; noticing 'shoulds' and 'musts' in our self-talk is a good indicator of when we are not being kind to ourselves.

Self-compassion can be defined as having three components (Neff 2011):

- Self-kindness
- Common humanity
- Mindfulness

In terms of self-kindness, this means the softening and understanding towards our mistakes, soothing and nurturing towards our own suffering when facing obstacles or struggles in life, and affording ourselves the same sympathy we would to a friend facing similar issues. We would do that with a sense of common humanity, a belief that 'we are all in the same boat'.

## Reflection point

- Consider for a moment, how many people are you aware of who have found life a struggle at one time or another and have needed support in some form to be able to cope?

When we struggle we often feel alone in our suffering and soldier on in isolation. This can lead to one feeling distanced from others and a sense that there is something wrong with us as we are struggling: 'Others seem to be okay – there's something wrong with me' – is that a familiar phrase? Judy, the student nurse, may continue to feel inadequate and weak, which will undoubtedly incur greater suffering and the potential for isolation. What one may argue once again is that feeling hurt and upset when witnessing another's distress should be perceived as normal rather than abnormal.

In fact, failure and imperfection is part and parcel of the human experience. Developing self-compassion is also helpful in developing our compassionate practice broadly, as the more self-compassionate we are, the more likely we are to show compassion to others (Neff and Pommier 2012), and indeed self-compassion can be helpful in coping with personal setbacks and challenges in life (Neff et al. 2005). Noticing 'shoulds' and 'musts' in our self-talk is key to accomplishing this. Now consider this from your own perspective in the following exercise.

## Working with the troubled self

In this exercise we will again spend a few moments engaging the compassionate self, feeling a sense of strength, wisdom and kindness. Remember, it is the intention and desire to be kind and helpful that is important.

Notice how your body feels, remember to focus on your facial expressions. When you feel that you have engaged with that part of you to some degree, try the following.

Imagine that you are watching a video of yourself, like watching a film. So you see yourself get up in the morning. Holding your position of kindness and compassion, watch yourself moving around in your room and then slowly getting on with your day. Notice how the person that you're watching (i.e. you) is troubled by self-critical feelings or thoughts about themselves, perhaps fears of their relationships with others or of being criticised, or fear of their feelings. Be in touch with the struggle of the person you're watching, but just hold your position of inner calmness and wisdom, looking out through the eyes of your compassionate self with the intention of being kind and helpful. If that sense of the compassionate self wanders, or you lose it in any way, just let the imagery fade, go back to your soothing breathing rhythm, your compassionate expression, sitting up straight in a confident posture, and begin again.

This exercise will help you to take a more objective view of your difficulties and also to begin developing your own intuitive wisdom and abilities to heal. Once we no longer fight with ourselves but become more accepting, and recognise the struggle that we can have in life (through no fault of our own), we might find it easier to gradually learn how to change.

## Support

The framework for this chapter is in response to current evidence surrounding dealing with stress and in response to research data of staff experiences in caring for patients at the end of life. Mindfulness or 'paying attention with intention' (Baer 2006) allows us to become aware of our habitual ways of thinking and acting, for example noticing negative thoughts and reactions towards oneself (Williams and Penman 2011). It is about stepping out from our familiar patterns of self-criticism and 'showing up' to experience end of life as it actually is, not what our minds tell us it is (Hayes et al. 2011). If, for example, we truly 'show up' and sit with the pain and fears of our patients as they approach the end of life, why wouldn't we notice sadness and anxiety in ourselves? Our minds have evolved to respond quickly to unwanted and aversive private content such as shame and embarrassment (Gilbert 2003), and so being mindful and open to our emotions and internal reactions requires practice and some courage.

Self-compassion, or the notion of being kind to ourselves (Neff 2010), is also not our natural default position. We may be familiar with feeling embarrassed and perhaps 'pathetic' at the way we reacted in a clinical situation, so one should consider the question 'What would you say to your sister or best friend if they talked to you about this?'. Unsurprisingly, you may come up with a different rhetoric that would undoubtedly be familiar with many of your colleagues, such as 'Don't be so hard on yourself'.

This speaks to the heart of self-compassion, allowing ourselves to have normal human reactions and feelings and affording ourselves the same care, respect and kindness that we afford to others (Tirch et al. 2014). Self-compassion training is vital to encourage this care for oneself.

## Values clarification

'Nursing values' are often referred to in healthcare literature (Sellman 2011) and are central to the NMC's code of conduct (2015) and Department of Health initiatives (DH 2012). The sense of a 'core value' to nursing practice is intrinsic within the role of a nurse, is well-established and has formed a central component of pre-registration nursing programmes since the outset (UK Central Council 1984; NMC 2010). What are perhaps less defined and attended to in nursing, however, are our personal values, what truly matters to us, what we stand for and what we want our lives to be about (Dahl et al. 2009). When applying for pre-registration training or a new nursing post one may speak quite eloquently about values and what nursing means to us, but on a day-to-day basis these thoughts may be at the back of our mind and replaced by the tasks in hand and the complexities of life. Revisiting what matters to us, as individuals, and clarifying our deeper-held principles and intentions is important and should be part of our reflective time. If we are not careful the NMC standards and proficiencies (NMC 2010, 2015) and professional guidelines for practice (RCN 2010) can become external rules to follow, whereas connecting to our own personal values and intentions on a regular basis may help us find the courage to make values-based behavioural choices even in difficult and aversive contexts (Dahl et al. 2009), such as busy wards or the intense emotional environment of a hospice.

 **Case scenario: Judy (part 3)**

Judy reflects on her experience and decides that she cannot continue to feel the way she does. Her guilt regarding the way she dealt with the distressed patient is overwhelming and affecting her emotionally, psychologically, socially and physically as she feels unwell now. She contacts a mentor from a previous placement and arranges to meet her. They sit and discuss the issues and her anxieties surrounding end of life care. The mentor identifies with the issues and confirms that she herself has similar worries and fears. Judy starts to feel less of a failure and that her feelings about the patient's distress are perhaps quite normal. Her mentor suggests that she look in the literature about end of life care and how to deal with difficult questions. She agrees to meet her again to discuss this further.

## Reflection points

- How beneficial do you think this was for Judy?
- How beneficial do you think it was for her mentor?
- Do you think it may change Judy's future practice?
- What benefit will there be to examining the literature?
- What do you think is happening here?

## Conclusion

Reflection on practice is beneficial for all involved in healthcare, allowing us to make sense of our experience, perhaps add theoretical components to aid understanding, and time to think about the whole situation in a constructive and analytical manner rather than simply responding as things happen (i.e. reflection in action) (Johns 2000). The NMC state that pre-registration education should result in competent reflexive practitioners (NMC 2010). The ability to reflect and make sense of end of life experience is crucial. For Judy, this could have a really positive impact on her own feelings about the way she acted and a beneficial effect for future patients in her care. Analysing the event, the care, the responses from those involved and how one felt about that experience can help both students and qualified staff. It can aid in the advancement of one's future practice by learning from situations that may not have gone so well, but also developing and building upon the positive aspects, for example, something said in response to a question or the skill demonstrated in symptom assessment or management.

## Conclusion

The requirement for high-quality end of life care delivery is undeniable (DH 2008); patients and their carers require support and need to know that the health and social care professionals are doing their absolute best to ensure that symptoms are managed and a holistic approach is adopted.

The degree of intimacy that may be required of the health and social care professional may, to some, be overwhelming and result in their own distress and exhaustion. Professionals need to be aware of the potential for this distress and know how, when and where to seek support. Without this, the care that the professional can expect to give may be less than adequate and the consequences of enduring distress on individuals may be severe and long-lasting to the point of irreversibility.

Helping students and other health and social care professionals to recognise this and give them the key skills to care for themselves and others should improve the health and wellbeing of staff and, as a result, the patient and their loved ones in their care.

# Suggested reading

Germer, C.K. and Neff, K.D. (2013) 'Self-compassion in clinical practice', *Journal of Clinical Psychology*, 69(8): 856–67.

Gilbert, P. (2009) *The Compassionate Mind: A New Approach to Facing the Challenges of Life*. London: Constable Robinson.

Neff, K.D. (2010) 'Review of the mindful path to self-compassion: Freeing yourself from destructive thoughts and emotions', *British Journal of Psychology*, 101: 179–81.

# References

Baer, R.A. (2006) *Mindfulness-based Treatment Approaches: A Clinician's Guide*. London: Elsevier.

Campbell, I.E., Larrivee, L., Field, P.A., Day, R.A. and Reutter, L. (1994) 'Learning to nurse in the clinical setting', *Journal of Advanced Nursing*, 20(6): 1125–31.

Chandler, C., Bodenhamer-Davis, E., Holden, J.M., Evenson, T. and Bratton, S. (2001) 'Enhancing personal wellness in counsellor trainees using bio-feedback: An exploratory study', *Behavioural Science*, 26: 67–89.

Cialkowska-Rysz, A. and Dzierzanowski, T. (2013) 'Personal fear of death affects the proper process of breaking bad news', *Archives of Medical Science*, 9(1): 127–31.

Clark, T. and Holmes, S. (2007) 'Fit for practice? An exploration of the development of newly qualified nurses using focus groups', *International Journal of Nursing Studies*, 44: 1210–20.

Curtis, K., Horton, K. and Smith, P. (2012) 'Student nurse socialisation in compassionate practice: A grounded theory study', *Nurse Education Today*, 32(7): 790–5.

Dahl, J.C., Plumb, J.C., Stewart, I. and Lundgren, T. (2009) *The Art and Science of Valuing in Psychotherapy: Helping Clients Discover, Explore, and Commit to Valued Action Using Acceptance and Commitment Therapy*. Oakland, CA: New Harbinger.

Dalai Lama (2002) *Open Heart: Practicing Compassion in Everyday Life*. London: Hachette.

Department of Health (2008) *End of Life Care Strategy Promoting High Quality Care for All Adults at the End of Life: Executive Summary*. London: DH. Available at: www.gov.uk/government/uploads/system/uploads/attachment_data/file/136443/EOLC_exec_summ.pdf (accessed 19.1.15).

Department of Health (2012) *Liberating the NHS: Developing the Healthcare Workforce From Design to Delivery*. London: DH. Available at: www.gov.uk/government/uploads/system/uploads/attachment_data/file/216421/dh_132087.pdf (accessed 19.1.15).

Francis, R. (2010) *The Mid Staffordshire NHS Foundation Trust Inquiry: Final Report of the Independent Inquiry into Care Provided by Mid Staffordshire NHS Foundation Trust*. Available at: www.midstaffspublicinquiry.com/report (accessed 19.1.15).

Germer, C.K. and Neff, K.D. (2013) 'Self-compassion in clinical practice', *Journal of Clinical Psychology*, 69(8): 856–67.

Gilbert, P. (2003) 'Evolution, social roles, and differences in shame and guilt', *Social Research: An International Quarterly of the Social Sciences*, 70: 1205–30.

Gilbert, P. (2009) *The Compassionate Mind: A New Approach to Facing the Challenges of Life*. London: Constable Robinson.

Gustin, L. and Wagner, L. (2013) 'The butterfly effect of caring – clinical nursing teachers' understanding of self-compassion as a source to compassionate care', *Scandinavian Journal of Caring Science*, 27(1): 175–83.

Hayes, S.C., Strosahl, K. and Wilson, K.G. (2011) *Acceptance and Commitment Therapy: The Process and Practice of Mindful Change*, 2nd edn. New York: Guilford Press.

Heffernan, M., Quinn Griffin, M.T., McNulty, S.R. and Fitzpatrick, J.J. (2010) 'Self-compassion and emotional intelligence in nurses', *International Journal of Nursing Practice*, 16: 366–73.

Higgins, G., Spencer, R.L. and Kane, R. (2010) 'A systematic review of the experiences and perceptions of the newly qualified nurse in the United Kingdom', *Nurse Education Today*, 30: 499–508.

Hopkinson, J., Hallett, C. and Luker, K. (2005) 'Everyday death: How do nurses cope with caring for dying people in hospital?', *International Journal of Nursing Studies*, 42: 125–33.

Irving, J.A., Dobkin, P.L. and Park, J. (2009) 'Cultivating mindfulness in health care professionals: A review of empirical studies of mindfulness-based stress reduction', *Complementary Therapies in Clinical Practice*, 15: 61–6.

Johns, C. (2000) *Becoming a Reflective Practitioner*, 2nd edn. Oxford: Blackwell.

Lillyman, S., Gutteridge, R. and Berridge, P. (2011) 'Using a storyboarding technique in the classroom to address end of life experiences in practice and engage student nurses in deeper reflection', *Nurse Education in Practice*, 11: 179–85.

Maben, J., Adams, M., Peccei, R., Murrells, T. and Robert, G. (2012) '"Poppets and parcels": The links between staff experience of work and acutely ill older peoples' experience of hospital care', *International Journal of Older People Nursing*, 7(2): 83–94.

Mackintosh, C. (2007) 'Protecting the self: A descriptive qualitative exploration of how registered nurses cope with working in surgical areas', *International Journal of Nursing Studies*, 44(6): 982–90.

McAllister, M. and McKinnon, J. (2009) 'The importance of teaching and learning resilience in the health disciplines: A critical review of the literature', *Nurse Education Today*, 29(4): 371–9.

Miller, N.M. and McGowen, R.K. (2000) 'The painful truth: Physicians are not invincible [review]', *Southern Medical Journal*, 93: 966–73.

National Health Service (2012) *Compassion in Practice: Nursing, Midwifery and Care Staff: Our Vision and Strategy*. Available at: www.england.nhs.uk/wp-content/uploads/2012/12/compassion-in-practice.pdf (accessed 4.6.15).

Neff, K.D. (2003) 'Development and validation of a scale to measure self-compassion', *Self and Identity*, 2: 223–50.

Neff, K.D. (2010) 'Review of the mindful path to self-compassion: Freeing yourself from destructive thoughts and emotions', *British Journal of Psychology*, 101: 179–81.

Neff, K.D. (2011) *Self-compassion*. New York: William Morrow.

Neff, K.D. and Pommier, E. (2012) 'The relationship between self-compassion and other-focused concern among college undergraduates, community adults, and practicing meditators', *Self and Identity*, 12(2): 160–76.

Neff, K.D., Hsieh, Y. and Dejitterat, K. (2005) 'Self-compassion, achievement goals, and coping with academic failure', *Self and Identity*, 4: 263–87.

Nursing and Midwifery Council (2010) *Standards for Pre-registration Education*. London: NMC.

Nursing and Midwifery Council (2015) *The Code: Professional Standards of Practice and Behaviour for Nurses and Midwives*. London: NMC.

Peters, L., Cant, R., Payne, S., O'Connor, M., McDermott, F., Hood, K., Morphet, J. and Shimoinaba, K. (2013) 'Emergency and palliative care nurses' levels of anxiety about death and coping with death: A questionnaire survey', *Australasian Emergency Nursing Journal*, 16: 152–9.

Royal College of Nursing (2008) *Nursing our Future: An RCN study into the Challenges Facing Today's Nursing Students in the UK*. London: RCN.

Royal College of Nursing (2010) *Principles of Nursing Practice: Principles and Measures Consultation*. London: RCN. Available at www.rcn.org.uk/__data/assets/pdf_file/0007/349549/003875.pdf (accessed 4.6.15).

Saunders, C. (1976) 'The challenge of terminal care', in T. Symington and R. Carter (eds), *The Scientific Foundations of Oncology*. London: Heinemann.

Schantz, M.L. (2007) 'Compassion: A concept analysis', *Nursing Forum*, 42(2): 48–55.

Sellman, D. (2011). *What Makes a Good Nurse: Why the Virtues are Important for Nurses*. London: Jessica Kingsley.

Tirch, D., Schoendorff, B. and Silberstein, L.R. (2014) *The ACT Practitioner's Guide to the Science of Compassion Tools for Fostering Psychological Flexibility*. Oakland, CA: New Harbinger.

United Kingdom Central Council (1984) *Annual Report of the Council 1983–1984*. London: UKCC.

van der Cingel, M. (2014) 'Compassion: The missing link in quality of care', *Nurse Education Today*, 34(9): 1253–7.

Whitehead, B., Owen, P., Holmes, D., Beddingham, E., Simmons, M., Henshaw, L., Barton, M. and Walker, C. (2013) 'Supporting newly qualified nurses in the UK: A systematic literature review', *Nurse Education Today*, 33(4): 370–7.

Williams, M. and Penman, D. (2011) *Mindfulness: A Practical Guide to Finding Peace in a Frantic World*. London: Piatkus.

# Index